Intensive Care of the Heart and Lungs

A TEXT FOR NURSES AND OTHER STAFF

J M Neutze   C T Möller

E A Harris   M P Horsburgh

M D Wilson

Foreword by
Sir Brian Barratt-Boyes

THIRD EDITION

Blackwell Scientific Publications
OXFORD LONDON EDINBURGH
BOSTON MELBOURNE

© 1972, 1975, 1982 by
Blackwell Scientific Publications
Editorial offices:
Osney Mead, Oxford OX2 0EL
8 John Street, London WC1N 2ES
9 Forrest Road, Edinburgh EH1 2QH
52 Beacon Street, Boston
    Massachusetts 02108 USA
99 Barry Street, Carlton
    Victoria 3053 Australia

First published 1972
Second Edition 1975
Revised Reprint 1978
Third Edition 1982

Set by Southline Press, Ferring,
W. Sussex
Printed and bound in Great Britain by
Billing and Sons Ltd., Guildford,
London, Oxford and Worcester

DISTRIBUTORS

USA
    Blackwell Mosby Book Distributors
    11830 Westline Industrial Drive
    St Louis, Missouri 63141

Canada
    Blackwell Mosby Book Distributors
    120 Melford Drive, Scarborough
    Ontario M1B 2X4

Australia
    Blackwell Scientific Book Distributors
    214 Berkeley Street, Carlton
    Victoria 3053

British Library
Cataloguing in Publication Data

Intensive care of heart and lungs: a text for
    nurses and other staff — 3rd ed.
    1. Cardiovascular disease nursing
    2. Coronary care units
    3. Respiratory organs — Diseases
    4. Critical care medicine
    I. Neutze, J. M.
    616.1′2   R674

ISBN 0–632–00925–X

Contents

Authors

J. M. Neutze MD FRACP
Physician, Cardiology Department, Green Lane Hospital, Auckland, New Zealand

C. T. Möller BSc (Hons) MB BCh FFA (SA)
Anaesthetist, Cardiothoracic Surgical Unit, Green Lane Hospital, Auckland, New Zealand

F. A. Harris MD PhD FRCP FRACP
Physician-in-Charge, Clinical Physiology Department, Green Lane Hospital, Auckland, New Zealand

Margaret P. Horsburgh SRN SCM BA
Nurse Tutor, Auckland Technical Institute, Auckland, New Zealand

Maree D. Wilson SRN
Nursing Supervisor, Cardiothoracic Surgical Unit, Green Lane Hospital, Auckland, New Zealand

Foreword
(to the first edition)

The publication of this monograph represents a milestone in cardiology and cardiac surgery at Green Lane Hospital, for it is the first book compiled by members of the unit. I hope and expect it to be the first of a series of monographs dealing with various facets of the diagnosis and treatment of cardiorespiratory disease, for the unit now has a wide experience in this field; an experience which encompasses many exciting developments in surgical heart disease from the neonate through to the elderly patient. It is perhaps a cogent reminder of the nature of New Zealand medical practice that Green Lane Hospital has not published a monograph or a textbook before 1972. This tardiness is the end result of a number of circumstances not readily apparent to our colleagues in the longer-established units in the United Kingdom and the United States, where there is a tradition of original contributions to medicine and facilities available to disseminate new knowledge. In contrast, New Zealand has concentrated in the past on sending its graduates to these countries to keep abreast with current developments. The staffing of New Zealand hospitals has been entirely orientated around patient care without regard for the additional staff and time required for researching and documenting their own contributions. At Green Lane Hospital the clinical load has been particularly onerous and the time is now ripe to pause and reflect and where possible document this large experience.

Good nursing care is a fundamental requirement of good hospital practice and it is therefore appropriate that this text should outline the principles and practice of intensive care room nursing. Dr. Harris and his co-authors are to be congratulated on producing a very readable, accurate and instructive book on this subject. The text has been based on lectures presented at the six-monthly post-certificate Course in Cardiothoracic Nursing which has been a popular feature of the nursing programme in this hospital since

1962, when the first surgical intensive care unit in New Zealand was established in the cardio-thoracic surgical ward at Green Lane Hospital. From its commencement this course has continued to attract 10 to 20 applicants from New Zealand and from overseas. I feel sure that future registrars and indeed all nurses engaged in intensive care will find this a valuable text, which will help them to understand the principles upon which the current management of the critically ill patient is based. I also suspect that junior medical staff engaged in this field will benefit from much of the text and will appreciate the clarity with which the complex subject matter is handled by the authors.

Nursing care has fortunately changed radically since the days of Florence Nightingale. Today's nurse not only has her responsibilities and duties more clearly defined; she also has much more to learn, particularly if she wishes to nurse the critically ill patient following open heart surgery. Although this type of nursing places considerable strain on personnel, the work is challenging, exciting and highly rewarding and the fear that intensive care nursing may be beyond her capabilities need not deter an intelligent, conscientious trained nurse. The text available in the following pages will go a long way towards increasing her confidence and improving the standards of intensive care.

Brian Barratt-Boyes   1972
KBE MB ChM FRACS FACS FRSNZ
Surgeon-in-Charge
Cardiothoracic Surgical Unit
Green Lane Hospital
Auckland, New Zealand

Preface

Only 3 years have passed since the last revision of this book, and the number of changes required is an indication of the remarkable changes in the field over this period. The sections on intensive care have been largely rewritten and the emphasis in some of the physiological sections modified to fit the changes.

As in the earlier editions, the book seeks primarily to be a 'Companion' for nurses in the Intensive Care Unit largely devoted to the care of patients after cardiac surgery. As such we have aimed to present the underlying physiological information required for an understanding of pathophysiologic changes and treatment. We have therefore not shunned difficult areas but sought to be accurate, even when a simplified account was necessary. Some sections of the book have been used increasingly by other staff, both paramedical and medical. The corpus of knowledge is the same for all staff and a volume of modest format can contain a surprising amount of practical detail. With this in mind, the content has been expanded somewhat, but not beyond the realm of the ICU nurse.

We have concentrated on those aspects having the greatest impact on management, and have tried to present sufficient detail to allow application of principles without becoming too involved in those minor aspects of technique which vary from one Unit to another. We crave the indulgence of the reader who finds too little detail in one area of his or her interest and too much in another.

Since the last revision Dr Harris has chosen to step down as the senior author, Dr Möller has replaced Drs Seelye and Simpson in the anaesthetic section, Ms Rickard has changed her name by marriage to Horsburgh, and Ms Wilson has joined the group of authors. We wish to thank Drs Patricia Clarkson, John Mercer, Robin Norris, Peter Doak, Jon Simcock, Warren Smith, Donald McCullough and Mr Brian Cornere for reviewing sections on the infant, ischaemic disease, renal disease, neurological assessment, arrhythmias and infection; Ms Barbara Williams, Patricia Taylor, Mary MacManus, Penelope Dunkley and Margaret Tucker the sections on ischaemia, infants and social problems; Mr Sydney Yarrow the section on pacing and Mr Ray Laurie the appendices on drug administration. Our thanks also go to Ms Donna Anderson and Messrs Ron Hart and Darryn Brown for the illustrations and photography and to Ms Margaret Wall and Joan Findlay for typing the manuscripts.

J. M. Neutze   *January 1982*
Green Lane Hospital, Auckland

Introduction

Advances in medical science and technology have brought about rapid and continuing change in medical and nursing attitudes to the care of sick people. Survival, improvement and even full recovery are now seen to be possible in acute and chronic illness which would have been thought hopeless a decade or so ago. The feasibility of complex surgical procedures, the advent of powerful new drugs and the development of mechanical aids to treatment have all presented new problems of management for which experience has had to lean increasingly on basic scientific principles; we have exchanged many dead certainties for living perplexities.

The intensive care unit, with its concentration of special facilities and trained staff for the treatment of selected patients at particular risk, has become a common feature of general hospitals everywhere. This unit may cater for any patient needing continuous attention, or it may be restricted to a single clinical speciality such as cardiac surgery or neurosurgery. In most such units, cardiovascular and respiratory deaths are the most probable ones, and cardiorespiratory intensive care is thus the cornerstone of treatment.

Intensive care is a great challenge and demands of a nurse, as of all staff, the highest qualities of character and competence. Whatever career a nurse may contemplate, a period spent in the Intensive Care Unit (ICU) will provide an invaluable experience.

Care of the patient in the ICU is a team effort and the nurse functions as an interdependent part of that team, collaborating with other staff to provide continuity of patient care.

The problem-solving approach, the nursing process, utilised in nursing practice is vital in the ICU where the patient's condition may change rapidly. The nursing process consists of a series of phases, or step-by-step actions, directed at problem solving. These phases are (1) assessment, or the collection, organisation and analysis of all information relevant to the individual's health status;

(2) planning an organised course of action to assist the individual in solving health problems; (3) intervening, or implementing the plan of action and (4) evaluating the effectiveness of the plan, and revising it as appropriate.

For problem-solving to be effective, nursing must have a theoretical and scientific base. The nurse in the ICU must have a thorough knowledge of normal human biology, of pathophysiology and of therapeutic measures including surgical techniques and pharmacological manipulations, as well as a knowledge of the social sciences allowing her or him to understand the patient as an individual. Accurate assessment, meticulous attention to detail, and adaptability are imperative in the ICU, since intensive care nursing presents unusual and often unexpected situations. The nurse must be able to evaluate and revise plans of action rapidly as the changing situation demands.

Many patients are admitted acutely to the ICU but ideally the ICU nurse will meet surgical patients preoperatively so that a full nursing history can be taken. The nurse must provide individualised patient care which includes involvement and consideration of the patient's family. Providing emotional support is as much a part of sound physiological care as are the overtly technical procedures of the ICU. Much can be done to allay the patient's anxiety by careful preoperative explanation of what the patient and family can expect, and a preliminary meeting with the nursing staff who will care for the patient. Although the patients in the ICU may be very ill and temporarily very dependent, they must be treated not as anonymous patients, but as individuals who can still participate to some degree in the direction of their own life. It is easy to forget that a patient who cannot speak because of the presence of a tracheostomy or who is paralysed, may be completely aware of the surroundings, and special care must be taken to explain procedures and to obtain the trust of the patient in such trying circumstances.

The problems of sensory overload and sleep deprivation for a patient surrounded as he or she is by a mass of equipment and by constant activity and noise may make a spell in the ICU a harrowing experience. The design of the Unit may help diminish these problems, but the nurse must constantly bear them in mind. Patients should be accorded as much privacy and consideration of their individual needs as is humanly possible.

Communication with relatives is an integral part of patient care, and is of special importance in the ICU. All staff should seek to provide full and regular explanations to relatives, visiting arrangements should be liberal and flexible, and somewhere quiet and private should be provided away from the main corridors and the tension of the ICU.

Moments of tension and emergency occur in the general wards of a hospital, but the ICU exists at a continuous level of either crisis or the expectation of it. Many nurses find the constant need for vigilance a great strain, and it is natural that feelings of inadequacy sometimes appear. These can be overcome if they are recognised by the nurses and their seniors and the basis discussed freely and sympathetically. Despite the difficulties and hazards mentioned — perhaps because of them — intensive care nursing can be immensely rewarding. It is true that a great deal of work may ultimately fail to save life, but even then the nurse should have learnt valuable lessons from the experience. The real prize is to see a patient restored, physically and mentally, to a happy, healthy life against tremendous odds, and to feel that one had some essential part in bringing this about.

This book seeks to contribute to the core of knowledge and understanding required for accurate assessment and intelligent treatment in the ICU. It aims to present principles, not to be an encyclopaedia of all relevant information or an instruction manual to replace in-service training. It will certainly have failed in its objectives if the reader does not have a desire for further information in some areas, and a willingness to search it out. A bibliography is included for reference to some aspects covered incompletely in this book.

I Anatomy and Physiology

1 Anatomy and Physiology

1 Body Chemistry

ELECTROLYTES AND ACID-BASE BALANCE

Unless the reader knows something of elementary chemistry, an account of electrolyte and acid-base physiology is mere mumbo-jumbo. Not all nurses have this knowledge, and it is thus necessary to clarify some basic points here.

Elements and atoms

A *chemical element* is a substance with characteristic properties (colour, specific gravity, chemical reactivity, etc.) which up to the present has not been shown to be composed of two or more different substances. An element may be a gas (e.g. oxygen), a liquid (e.g. mercury) or a solid (e.g. carbon).

An *atom* is the smallest particle of an element which retains the distinctive properties of that element. It is very small indeed, far beyond the limits of even the most powerful microscope. One milligram (mg) of an element contains millions of atoms.

Atomic weight. Atoms of different elements differ from each other in weight. The lightest is the atom of hydrogen, the weight of

Table 1 Atomic weights (to the nearest 0·5).

Element	Atomic weight	Symbol	Element	Atomic weight	Symbol
Hydrogen	1·0	H	Sulphur	32·0	S
Carbon	12·0	C	Chlorine	35·5	Cl
Nitrogen	14·0	N	Potassium	39·0	K
Oxygen	16·0	O	Calcium	40·0	Ca
Sodium	23·0	Na	Iron	56·0	Fe
Magnesium	24·0	Mg	Mercury	200·5	Hg
Phosphorus	31·0	P			

which is assigned the value 1. An oxygen atom weighs 16 times as much, and its atomic weight is therefore 16. These are special weight units, not mg or any other conventional unit of weight; they merely give the relative weights of the different atoms. Some useful atomic weights are given in Table 1.

Molecules, compounds and mixtures

Two or more atoms of any kind which are bound together in a particular way constitute a *molecule*. The atoms may be of the same kind; for instance oxygen ordinarily exists as molecules, each containing two atoms, and this is the form in which oxygen enters into chemical reactions; this is why we write 'O_2' for oxygen. Or a molecule may consist of atoms of different kinds; for example, the magnesium sulphate molecule has one magnesium, one sulphur and four oxygen atoms, and is written $MgSO_4$. A substance like this, consisting of molecules constructed from dissimilar atoms, is called a *compound*. The molecule is the smallest particle of any compound which retains the properties of that compound. It can be split up into smaller particles, but these are quite different from the compound; in the above example we should end up with magnesium, sulphur and oxygen, which are quite different from magnesium, sulphate. This pinpoints the differences between a compound and a *mixture*. The constituents of a mixture may be present in any proportion to each other, whereas the elements of a particular compound are present in fixed proportions. The properties of a mixture are those of its individual constituents; a compound has quite different properties from any of its component elements. The constituents of a mixture can be separated more or less easily; those of a compound are bound to (or *combined with*) each other by powerful forces which keep the molecule together and special means are needed to separate them.

The *molecular weight* of a compound (or of an element which exists in the form of molecules) is simply the sum of the atomic weights of the atoms of which its molecules are composed.

Ionization and electrolysis

The molecules of many water-soluble compounds have the property, when in solution, of splitting into two or more parts called *ions*.

The essential feature of an ion is that it is electrically charged. The charge may be positive or negative and an ion may have one, two or three charges. The important ions and their symbols are shown in Table 2.

Table 2 Some common ions.

Cations		Anions	
Hydrogen	H^+	Chloride	Cl^-
Sodium	Na^+	Sulphate	SO_4^{--}
Potassium	K^+	Phosphate	PO_4^{---}
Magnesium	Mg^{++}	Bicarbonate	HCO_3^-
Calcium	Ca^{++}		

The process of ionization occurs as soon as the ionizable compound is dissolved in water, and the ions remain separate only in the presence of water. Examples of ionization are the following:

$$KCl \rightleftharpoons K^+ + Cl^-$$
potassium chloride   potassium ion   chloride ion
$$CaCl_2 \rightleftharpoons Ca^{++} + 2Cl^-$$
calcium chloride   calcium ion   two chloride ions

These changes are reversible, as shown by the double arrows.

If two electrodes are immersed in a solution of an ionizable compound and then connected to the poles of a battery, an electric current flows through the solution. Pure water conducts electricity very badly, but the presence in it of ions allows the current to pass freely. The ions themselves move through the solution, positively charged ones to the negative electrode or cathode, and negatively charged ones to the positive electrode or anode. The positive and negative ions are thus called *cations* and *anions* respectively. A compound which ionizes, and allows current to pass through a solution of it, is called an *electrolyte*.

One ion has special properties and importance. This is the hydrogen ion (H^+), the concentration of which in a solution determines the degree of acidity of the solution. Water itself contains a very low concentration of H^+ and is taken as neutral. The addition of more hydrogen ion (as by adding hydrochloric acid, HCl, which ionizes into H^+ and Cl^-) makes the solution acid. The removal of some hydrogen ions from water makes it alkaline. Acidity and alkalinity are measured in pH units. A high H^+ concentration, and therefore acidity, goes with a low pH value. A low H^+ concentration, and therefore alkalinity, goes with a high pH. Water has a pH of 7·0. Blood has a pH of about 7·4, and is therefore slightly alkaline compared with water. In *acidosis* pH may be as low as 6·9; in *alkalosis* pH may be as high as 7·8.

Units of weight, volume and concentration

In Sèvres, France, is a Standard Kilogram (kg) weight on which the metric weight system is based. Successive divisions by 1000 give:

1 gram (g)	= 1/1000 kg
1 milligram (mg)	= 1/1000 g
1 microgram (μg)	= 1/1000 mg
1 nanogram (ng)	= 1/1000 μg

The volume of 1 kg of pure water at 4°C is defined as a litre (l). Dividing again by 1000, we have

1 millilitre (ml)	= 1/1000 l
1 microlitre (μl)	= 1/1000 ml

1 ml, for all practical purposes, is the same as 1 cubic centimetre (cc).

Metric units should always be used, but for comparison with Imperial Units we have 1 pint = 0·568 l = 568 ml.

Concentration describes the amount of a constituent of a mixture present in a given quantity of the mixture. For dissolved solids we can say 'so many mg (or g, or kg) per ml (or 100 ml, or l) of the solution'. The term '5 per cent glucose' implies a concentration of 5 g of glucose per 100 ml of solution. The common unit in work with body fluids is 'mg per 100 ml' because this gives a sensible number for most dissolved substances in the body.

Moles, millimoles, equivalents and milliequivalents

Suppose we have in a shopping basket 1 lb of cherries, 1 lb of plums, 1 lb of apples and 1 lb of peaches. We cannot say, from this information, how many of each type of fruit we have, or even what proportion they bear to each other. On the other hand, if we know the weights of 1 cherry, 1 plum, 1 apple and 1 peach we could calculate the numbers of each in our basket.

The actions of ions or atoms or molecules in the body are much more affected by how many of them are available than by how much they weigh. For this reason it is a great convenience to express their concentrations in a way which bears a direct relation to the numbers of ions and atoms and molecules present. An example will help to make this clear. One litre of normal serum contains 3220 mg of sodium and 175·5 mg of potassium. For every 1 mg of potassium there are thus 3220/175·5, or 18·3 mg of sodium. This is the relationship by weight between these two elements. But from Table 1 we know that each atom (or ion) of potassium is heavier than an atom (or ion) of sodium, by a factor of 39/23, and it is evident that for every *ion* of potassium there must be more sodium ions than the proportion indicated on the basis of weight. How can we express the relative numbers of these ions present per litre?

The answer is to use the system of *equivalent weights*. The atomic (and ionic) weight of sodium is 23, and one equivalent of sodium is defined as 23 grams; one milliequivalent weighs 1/1000 of this, or 23 mg. Similarly, 1 milliequivalent of potassium weighs 39 mg. Using the example given above, 3220 mg of sodium contain 3220/23, or 140 mEq, and 175·5 mg of potassium contain 175·5/39 or 4·5 mEq. We thus express the concentrations of these ions as 140 and 4·5 mEq/l respectively. Since we have taken the atomic (or ionic) weight into account, these concentrations provide a true estimate of the relative numbers of each ion present; the proportion is 140 of sodium to 4·5 of potassium, or a ration of 31 to 1 approximately. This is almost twice the proportion suggested by the relative gross weights—18·3 as calculated above.

As shown in Table 2, some ions have more than one electrical charge. An ion with two charges is chemically equivalent to two ions with one charge, and in calculating the equivalent weight of such a *divalent* ion we must divide its atomic (or ionic) weight by 2. A *trivalent* ion such as phosphate, with 3 charges, must have its ionic weight divided by 3. The ions we have to deal with most commonly are, however, *monovalent* like sodium and potassium, and in this case the ionic weight equals the equivalent weight.

Summarizing, to find the equivalent weight of an ion we look up its *ionic weight* in Table 1 and divide this by its *valency*, shown in

Table 2 by the number of charges. The answer, in grams is 1 equivalent and, in milligrams, 1 milliequivalent (mEq).

Many molecules do not ionize in solution, e.g. glucose and urea. In these cases the terms mole (mol) or millimole (mmol) are applied. One mol is simply the molecular weight in grams, and 1 mmol the molecular weight in milligrams. These units, again, give us a direct estimate of the relative numbers of molecules in solution. Since these molecules do not ionize, valency does not enter into the calculation.

SI units are now standard in many countries. According to this system Eq and mEq are no longer used and are replaced by mol and mmol for all substances, whether ionized or not. 1 mmol of a univalent ion is the same as 1 mEq, of a divalent ion 2 mEq, and so on. The SI units are used in this book.

Osmotic pressure

The cells of the body are enclosed by membranes through which water passes freely. Dissolved substances also pass through, but with differing degrees of difficulty so that some are virtually confined to one side of the membrane. A membrane which behaves like this is called *semipermeable*, since water and some dissolved compounds can pass through it whereas others cannot.

In Fig. 1 (1) a semipermeable membrane separates two chambers each containing sodium chloride solution of the same concentration. To side A is added albumin, which cannot pass through the membrane. Solution A is now more concentrated, in terms of dissolved particles, than solution B. Water passes from B to A until B and A are of more equal concentration. In the process level A rises and level B falls (2), establishing a pressure head A'B' between the two chambers. The more concentrated the albumin originally, the greater the pressure A'B'. This is called the *osmotic pressure* of the protein solution. There is a redistribution of Na^+ and Cl^- across the membrane, but this need not concern us. The point to note is that *whenever there is a rise in concentration of a substance on one side of a membrane which is not permeable to it, water is attracted towards the side containing this substance. If its concentration falls, water moves in the opposite direction.*

It is by the operation of osmotic forces that the distribution of body water is regulated. The walls of blood vessels are impermeable

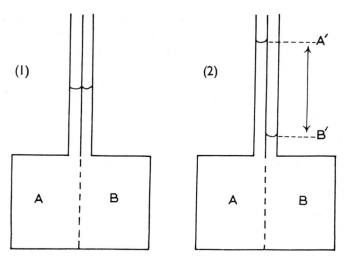

Fig. 1 Osmotic pressure. Chambers A and B are separated by semi-permeable membrane. The left-hand diagram shows equal pressure, when A and B are filled with solutions which can diffuse through the membrane. In the right-hand diagram a non-diffusible solute, such as protein, has been added to chamber A. Water passes from B to A, lowering pressure B and raising pressure A. The height A' B' is a measure of the osmotic pressure of the solution in A.

to plasma proteins but allow water and electrolytes, as well as small molecules like glucose and urea, to pass through. Most cells other than those lining capillaries are impermeable also to sodium and potassium under normal conditions.

Body water

The water content of the body is 60–70 per cent by weight. In an average adult, this amounts to 42 kg, and thus 42 l, of water. This water is partly inside and partly outside cells, and is described as *intracellular* or *extracellular*. The extracellular water is partly inside and partly outside the circulation, and is described as *intravascular* or *extravascular*. These divisions or 'compartments' of body water are very important, because their chemical compositions are very different and the they behave in many ways independently. Their main characteristics are shown in Table 3.

It is obvious from Table 3 that there cannot be free interchange of all substances from one compartment to another, otherwise their concentrations would be the same. The walls of capillary blood-vessels (which separate plasma from the rest of the ECF) and the cell membranes (which separate ECF and ICF) act indeed as semipermeable membranes. The passage of water from one compartment to another is therefore governed by the concentrations of those substances to which the membranes are impermeable (p. 8). In the case of the capillary walls, protein is the only factor involved. In the case of cell membranes, the extracellular Na^+ concentration is an important factor because in effect the cell membrane is, under normal conditions, impermeable to it. The concentration of K^+ and of protein inside the cells are also presumably important for the same reason, but since they are not easily measured we know little about the part they play.

The operation of osmotic forces can be illustrated by the effects of intravenous infusion of the three main fluids we use—plasma, isotonic saline and 5 per cent glucose.

1 *Plasma.* The infused plasma has a protein concentration which is the same as that of the patient's plasma, and there is thus no change in this after the infusion. The infused protein cannot pass through

Table 3 Body fluid composition.

	Intracellular fluid	Extracellular fluid	
Volume (l)	27	13	Intravascular 3 Extravascular ('interstitial') 10
Sodium (mmol per l)	10	140	
Potassium (mmol per l)	150	5	
Chloride (mmol per l)	10	100	

The following points should be noted:
1 The intravascular volume of 3 l is that of blood water only; the solids of the blood make up the remaining 2 l of blood volume.
2 Extracellular fluid (ECF) contains a lot of Na^+ and Cl^- but little K^+.
3 Intracellular fluid (ICF) contains a lot of K^+ but little Na^+ or Cl^-.
4 Protein is plentiful in cells and in intravascular fluid (plasma) but is almost absent from extravascular, extracellular fluid.
5 The remaining 2 l of water (to make up 42 l) are contained in bowel, bladder, etc.

the capillary wall. The osmotic conditions are unchanged, and *all the infused plasma water stays in the blood vessels*. The blood volume therefore increases but the extravascular ECF and the ICF volumes are unaltered. Other solutions of large molecules which cannot escape from the capillaries behave in the same way (haemaccel, dextran, albumin, stable plasma protein solution—SPPS).

2 *Isotonic sodium chloride solution*. This has a sodium concentration of 150 mmol per l, similar to that of the ECF. (The term 'normal saline' is commonly used as a synonym for isotonic sodium chloride solution. This usage is not recommended, since the term 'normal' means something quite different in chemistry.) The infused water and sodium chloride first enter the plasma and dilute the plasma protein. Water therefore passes out of the plasma and, since the capillaries are completely permeable to Na^+ and Cl^-, these ions pass out too. Eventually *the infused water and salt are evenly distributed throughout the ECF*, and since the latter's Na^+ concentration is the same as before there will be no tendency for water to pass into or out of the cells. The plasma protein concentration ends by being a little lower than it was, but not nearly as low as it would have been had the infused water all stayed in the circulation.

3 *5 per cent glucose (dextrose) solution*. Glucose passes through the capillary walls freely, and the initial effects are therefore as in 2 above. But the cell membrane is also freely permeable to glucose (provided that insulin is present), and unlike 2 the extracellular Na^+ has been diluted by the sodium-free infusion. Osmotic forces at the cell membrane are thus reduced, and water and glucose therefore pass into the cells. Eventually *the infused water and glucose are evenly distributed throughout the body water, both ECF and ICF*. Note that this result depends upon the cell membrane's permeability to glucose. Another sugar, mannitol, passes into the cell only with difficulty, and thus exerts an osmotic effect of its own; the infused water, in this case, is largely confined to the ECF.

With this background, it is easy to predict what will happen when other solutions are infused. A common one is one-fifth isotonic saline, 4·2 per cent glucose solution. One litre of this is equivalent to 1/5 l of isotonic saline plus 4/5 l of 5·25 per cent glucose solution. The 200 ml of isotonic saline stays in the ECF while the remaining 800 ml is distributed throughout the body water.

It will also readily be understood why the margin of safety differs for the various types of infusion. Plasma is infused into a potential water compartment of only 3 l, isotonic saline 13 l and glucose solution 40 l. It is thus easiest to overload the circulation with plasma and least easy to overload with glucose solution.

Regulation of body water

The total body water and its distribution is normally kept remarkably constant, despite wide fluctuations in intake and losses. Two mechanisms work together to maintain this balance.

1 *Aldosterone* is a hormone secreted by the cortex of the suprarenal gland. Its secretion is mainly controlled by a reflex mechanism. The reflex arises in the wall of the right atrium, and elsewhere in the cardiovascular system, in response to underfilling of the circulation. The response to this is the secretion of aldosterone which increases reabsorption of Na in the distal tubules of the kidneys (p. 93). Sodium is therefore retained, while H^+ and K^+ are lost to the body; K^+ depletion and alkalosis thus follow. Retention of Na^+ increases its concentration in ECF and this triggers the ADH mechanism described below. Aldosterone is secreted in increased amounts in haemorrhagic shock because of the decrease in blood volume. It also increases whenever cardiac output is reduced, and is partly responsible for the sodium retention and potassium loss which characterize congestive cardiac failure.

2 *Antidiuretic hormone* (ADH) is secreted by the posterior lobe of the pituitary gland. Its secretion is regulated by specialized nerve cells called *osmoreceptors* which lie near the pituitary gland at the base of the brain. These cells are sensitive to changes in concentration of Na^+ in ECF. When Na^+ concentration rises, ADH secretion increases. ADH acts by increasing the reabsorption of water, from the lumen of the distal and collecting tubules, to the ECF (p. 95); urinary volume therefore falls and water retention occurs. This in turn causes the concentration of ECF to return to normal.

The interaction of these two control mechanisms explains why primary gain or loss of sodium is almost always accompanied by gain or loss of water. Primary gain or loss of water, however, is not directly linked with a similar gain or loss of sodium. For example, in cardiac failure, restriction of Na^+ and promotion of Na^+ loss by diuretics inevitably result in the loss of water too; but restriction of water does not promote the excretion of Na^+.

Disorders of water and electrolyte balance

Patients in an ICU are particularly at risk of developing excess or deficiency of water and electrolytes. The need to restrict intake, for several days, to the intravenous route, the frequent association of either temporary or permanent renal impairment, the metabolic and circulatory consequence of cardiac failure and surgical trauma, and the often poor nutritional state of the patient before admission, make necessary continuous assessment and control of water and electrolyte balance. This is especially true when the patient is an infant or small child.

An important aim of intravenous therapy is to meet the needs of the individual patient with respect to blood volume, sodium, potassium and water requirements, and these vary widely from case to case. They are assessed partly from the previous history, partly from analyses of serum and partly from balance studies. The latter are important in any patient needing more than a couple of days' treatment. To carry out a balance study it is essential to have exact information about the volume and electrolyte content of all intake (by whatever route) and of all urine excreted. It usually falls to the nursing staff to record these and make accurately timed collections of urine.

Potassium depletion must be briefly mentioned. In the ICU it is often met because

1   Cardiac failure alone causes K^+ depletion.
2   Treatment with diuretics increases the loss of K^+ in the urine (p. 108).
3   K^+ loss is part of the metabolic response to surgical and other stress (p. 24).
4   IPPV increases K^+ loss via aldosterone release (p. 223).
5   Excessive gastrointestinal losses often occur.

K^+ depletion can seldom be detected simply by finding a low serum K^+ concentration. Very little of the total body K^+ is held in the ECF — about 60 mmol out of a total of 3000–4000 mmol. A fall in serum K^+ from 4·5 to 2·5 mmol per l means a loss to the ECF of only 26 mmol of K^+. Important K^+ depletion amounts to 1000 mmol or more, and it is obvious that this must come out of the cells. Moreover, the serum K^+ level may be, and very often is, normal in the presence of K^+ depletion. We depend for diagnosis, therefore upon (a) an awareness of the possibility of K^+ depletion in a given situation, and (b) the results of electrolyte balance studies.

The effects of K^+ depletion are:

1   Cardiac arrhythmias (extrasystoles, ectopic tachycardia, ventricular fibrillation) especially when the patient is digitalized.

2   Paralytic ileus due to suppression of intestinal peristalsis.

3   Weakness and confusion.

Potassium may be given orally or intravenously as potassium chloride (KCl). Orally it tends to cause vomiting unless in 'slow release' form; intravenously it causes severe pain if infused too rapidly. The rate of infusion will depend upon the requirements but should not usually exceed 5 mmol per hour. *Intravenous potassium may cause cardiac arrest and must be given with great care*. The entry of K^+ into cells is promoted by glucose and insulin, and these may need to be given at the same time.

Acids and bases

An *acid* is a substance which in solution ionizes to form hydrogen ions (p. 5). A *base* is a substance which has the property of combining with hydrogen ions and thus reducing concentration of free H^+.

The ionizable products of metabolism are almost all acidic.

1   *Carbon dioxide* is not itself acidic, but combines with water to form carbonic acid.

$$CO_2 \qquad + \qquad H_2O \qquad \rightleftharpoons \qquad H_2CO_3$$

Carbon dioxide   Water   Carbonic acid

Carbonic acid ionizes in solution, as follows

$$H_2CO_3 \qquad \rightleftharpoons \qquad H^+ \qquad + \qquad HCO_3^-$$

Carbonic acid   Hydrogen ion   Bicarbonate ion

Carbon dioxide is thus potentially an acid.

2   The metabolism of fats produces a series of acids. Normally these are further metabolized to CO_2 and water, but in diabetic acidosis they accumulate. *Aceto-acetic acid* is an example of this group.

3   The phosphorus and sulphur in fats and proteins give rise to *phosphoric* and *sulphuric* acids.

4 Carbohydrate metabolism yields *pyruvic* and *lactic acids*. Normally these are further metabolized to CO_2 and water, but in the absence of oxygen this cannot happen. Thus hypoxia causes an increase in these acids.

Acid-base balance

An accumulation of hydrogen ions in the body is called an *acidosis*, and depletion of hydrogen ions is called *alkalosis*. Most laboratories measure the hydrogen ion concentration in pH units (p. 6). The pH depends on the balance of acids and bases. This relationship is described mathematically by the Henderson-Hasselbalch equation.;

$$pH = pK + \text{Log} \ \frac{[HCO_3^-]}{\alpha P_{CO_2}}$$

where pK is a constant (6·1) and α another constant (the solubility of CO_2 in plasma). A schematic model of the relationship is illustrated in Fig. 2.

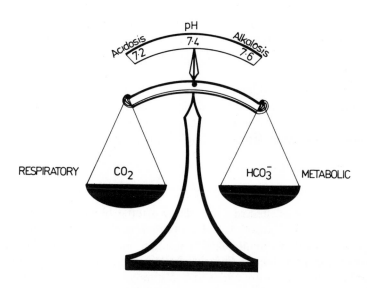

Fig. 2 The 'acid-base balance'.

It is clear that the pH will be altered by changes of either the P_{CO_2} or the bicarbonate ion concentration. An *acidosis* (pH below 7·4) will be caused by an *increase* in the P_{CO_2} or by a *decrease* in the bicarbonate ion concentration. Conversely, *alkalosis* (pH above 7·4) will result from a *decreased* P_{CO_2} or an *increased* concentration of bicarbonate ions.

It is also clear that, once upset, the balance can be restored either by *correction* on the abnormal side or by *compensation* on the other side.

'Respiratory' and 'metabolic' acidosis

The production of increased amounts of acids, or failure to excrete them properly, leads to an acidosis. When acidosis is due to a failure to excrete CO_2 it is called *respiratory acidosis* because the lungs are the only pathway through which CO_2 can be eliminated. Acidosis due to any other acid is called *metabolic acidosis*. Examples of metabolic acidosis are:

Ketoacidosis seen in diabetes (p. 199), phosphoric and sulphuric acidosis seen in renal failure and lactic acidosis which occurs in hypoxia.

These metabolic acids decrease the plasma bicarbonate ion concentration by reacting with bicarbonate.

$$H^+ + HCO_3^- = H_2CO_3$$

The amount by which the plasma bicarbonate ion concentration is decreased is called the *base deficit* which is an assessment of the number of hydrogen ions that have reacted in this way. In most laboratories a base deficit is reported as a negative *base excess* (e.g. BE − 7).

Recognition of acidosis

In both types of acidosis, the pH of arterial blood is below the normal range (7·36–7·42). Respiratory acidosis, by definition (p. 87), is due to inadequate ventilation and is accompanied by hypercapnia. In metabolic acidosis, hyperventilation is the most striking clinical feature and is due to stimulation of the respiratory centre (p. 75). This hyperventilation causes a compensatory reduction in the P_{CO_2} so that the pH tends towards normal. Arterial

P_{CO_2} is high in respiratory acidosis but low in metabolic acidosis with respiratory compensation.

In a given case acidosis may be of both 'respiratory' and 'metabolic' origin, and arterial blood analysis is essential to assess the position and follow progress.

Consequences of acidosis. Cardiac arrhythmias are less easily treated in the presence of acidosis, and hypoxia is less well tolerated. In general it is desirable to correct any appreciable degree of acidosis since, even if it is relatively mild, a further rapid increase in acidosis may have disastrous consequences.

Treatment of acidosis. **1** *Respiratory acidosis* is dealt with by increasing ventilation, if necessary by mechanical means (IPPV, p. 250).
2 *Metabolic acidosis* calls for treatment of its cause (hypoxia, diabetes, renal failure), and for correction of the acidosis itself by the administration of sodium bicarbonate ($NaHCO_3$). This supplies bicarbonate ions (HCO_3^-) which combine with H^+ to form carbonic acid (H_2CO_3). This in turn supplies CO_2 which is excreted by the lungs. This action of $NaHCO_3$ thus depends upon the efficacy of ventilation, and is of no value in respiratory acidosis.

Another substance which has been used to treat acidosis is tris-hydroxymethyl—aminomethane (abbreviated THAM). This penetrates into cells better than bicarbonate and so neutralizes cellular acidosis more effectively. However, THAM is toxic (hypoglycaemia and electrolyte disturbances) and only a limited amount of it can be given safely (0·3 mol in 1 hour, 0·6 mol in 12 hours).

Alkalosis

This is less often a problem in the ICU but may occur after prolonged vomiting, after gross overventilation, in potassium depletion and after excessive infusion of bicarbonate. It is usually sufficient to eliminate its cause. Tetany or convulsions may occur as a result of alkalosis, owing to a reduction in ionized calcium in the body fluids (serum total calcium concentration is unchanged). The injection of calcium chloride or gluconate will usually deal with this complication until the alkalosis can be corrected.

An approach to the interpretation of laboratory acid-base results

Consider this example:

pH 7·35
P_{CO_2} 4·3 kPa (32 mmHg)
BE −7 mmol per l

1 Look at the pH and decide if it indicates acidosis or alkalosis. The pH of 7·35 in the example indicates acidosis.
2 Look at the P_{CO_2} and BE. Decide which explains the pH. In the example the acidosis is explained by the BE of −7 indicating that the acidosis is *metabolic* in origin. If both the P_{CO_2} and BE explain the pH, a combined respiratory and metabolic derangement is present.
3 Look at the third component to decide if there is any compensation. The example shows a lower than normal P_{CO_2} indicating respiratory compensation for the metabolic acidosis.

One concludes that the example indicates a metabolic acidosis with respiratory compensation. Examination of the patient would confirm mild hyperventilation and may reveal the cause of the metabolic acidosis. It must be stressed that the clinical picture is most important and should be the first consideration in the interpretation of any laboratory results.

More examples of laboratory results are given in Table 4. In each case the bicarboate ion concentration is included as the BE is not reported by all laboratories.

METABOLISM

Metabolism is the term used to describe all the chemical reactions which occur in the body. We may picture the body as a chemical factory which takes in raw materials, processes these in various ways to meet different needs, and discharges waste products for which no use can be found. The body takes in substances as food (*ingestion*), deals with these chemically (*utilization*) at a certain rate appropriate to need (*metabolic rate*), *stores* some of the products for use in times of shortage and *excretes* what it cannot use.

Generally speaking there are two types of chemical reaction:

Table 4 Examples of various acid-base abnormalities.

	Respiratory		Metabolic	
	Alkalosis	Acidosis	Alkalosis	Acidosis
Uncompensated				
pH	7·50	7·29	7·50	7·29
P_{CO_2} kPa(mmHg)	4·0(30)	7·3(55)	5·5(41)	5·3(40)
HCO_3^- mmol per l	23	25	32	19
BE mmol per l	+1	−1	+8	−7
Compensated				
pH	7·41	7·38	7·44	7·35
P_{CO_2} kPa(mmHg)	4·0(30)	7·3(55)	6·7(50)	4·3(32)
HCO_3^- mmol per l	19	31	33	17
BE mmol per l	−4	+6	+8	−7

	Combined respiratory and metabolic	
	Alkalosis	Acidosis
pH	7·59	7·21
P_{CO_2} kPa(mmHg)	4·0(30)	7·3(55)
HCO_3^- mmol per l	29	21
BE mmol per l	+8	−7

1 Complex molecules are broken down into simpler, smaller ones. This is termed *catabolism* and it is useful in two ways: (a) it furnishes simple building blocks for the second type of reaction, **2**, and (b) it liberates energy (see below) which is essential for all living processes.

2 Small, relatively simple molecules, either ingested or produced by catabolism, are built up into bigger, more complex molecules different from the molecules from which the 'building blocks' originally came. This process is called *anabolism* and it is essential for the formation of the specific structural materials which are different from one species to another. However, the body cannot make everything it needs from the simplest materials. Some quite complex substances have to be provided, e.g. many amino-acids, some fats and the vitamins. Most anabolic reactions do not liberate energy but on the contrary they consume it.

Energy production and utilization

Energy is best defined as the capacity to do work, and (like work) it may take several forms which are interchangeable. The body needs chemical energy to drive anabolic reactions, thermal energy to maintain body temperature, electrical energy to excite and transmit nervous impulses and contractions of muscle, and mechanical energy for exercise. All these forms of energy are measured in units of their thermal energy equivalent. One unit is the Calorie (Cal), the amount of heat required to raise the temperature of 1 kg of water by 1 degree centigrade. The SI unit of heat is the kilojoule (kJ); 1 Cal equals 4·184 kJ.

Since all energy produced by the body is derived from the oxidation of foodstuffs, it is of interest to know the energy-value of different foods. The metabolism of 1 g of fat produces about 9 Cal, and that of 1 g of carbohydrate and 1 g of protein about 4 Cal each. A daily diet consisting of 80 g of protein, 400 g of carbohydrate and 120 g of fat would therefore supply 3000 Cal. The 'calorie-requirement' depends upon the amount of exercise taken, but even at complete rest energy is needed; this *basal metabolic rate* is about 1500 Cal per day for an average adult. A moderately active person needs 2500 Cal daily, a heavy manual worker 4000 Cal.

Food taken in excess of energy expenditure is mainly stored as fat. When the diet does not meet the calorie-requirements the fat stores are used, and when these are depleted the body protein is broken down and used for energy, rather as a man might use his furniture as firewood when no other fuel can be had. Any available fat, or especially carbohydrate, will be consumed in preference to body protein, and these foodstuffs are therefore termed 'protein sparers'. Protein and energy losses in some hospitalized patients are summarized in Appendix 4.

Metabolism of foodstuffs

A general knowledge of metabolic pathways is important as a background for work in the ICU and for an understanding of the metabolic effects of surgical operations.

Carbohydrates

These are eaten as sugars and starches, which are largely built up from simple 6-carbon molecules such as glucose, $C_6H_{12}O_6$. In the gut these *polysaccharides* are broken down to their 6-carbon units and absorbed in this form. In the liver, these units are re-built into a different polysaccharide called *glycogen* which is stored there. Liver glycogen is a reservoir which supplies glucose to the blood according to need. Unless replenished from dietary carbohydrate, liver glycogen lasts only 10 hours.

The muscles also have a store of glycogen, available 'on the spot' to supply glucose for muscle contraction. Muscle glycogen is replenished from the glucose in the blood. Other tissues do not contain stores of glycogen, but depend on minute-to-minute supply of glucose from the blood.

The concentration of glucose in the blood therefore depends upon the following factors:

Increasing blood glucose
1 Absorption of glucose from the small intestine.
2 Breakdown of glycogen in the liver, favoured by a low blood sugar and by stimulation of sympathetic nerves to the liver or infusion of adrenaline or isoprenaline (p. 32).
3 The activity of cortisol (p. 135) and related steroids, which antagonize insulin.

Reducing blood glucose
4 Formation of glycogen in the liver, favoured by insulin.
5 Entry of glucose into cells, favoured by insulin.
6 Consumption of glucose in the muscles, which is rapid during heavy exercise. Muscle glycogen is used up in about 4 to 8 hours of heavy exercise and the blood glucose concentration then begins to fall.

The utilization of glucose can be described by the equation
$$C_6H_{12}O_6 \ + \ 6O_2 \ \rightarrow \ 6CO_2 \ + \ 6H_2O$$
glucose   oxygen   carbon dioxide   water

Energy is liberated by this reaction. In the absence of O_2, a much smaller amount of energy is available from another reaction:

$$C_6H_{12}O_6 \ \rightarrow \ 2C_3H_6O_3$$
glucose   lactic acid

This provides enough energy to allow cells to survive short periods
of anoxia. In hypoxia, therefore, lactic acid appears in the cells and
blood.

Fats

These form several large groups of substances, which have in common a high carbon content and relatively low oxygen content.
Weight for weight, therefore, they are more 'combustible' than
carbohydrates, and are indeed a rich source of energy. In addition,
the body fat represents the biggest energy reserve. Fats are oxidized
to carbon dioxide and water with the release of energy. For this to
proceed efficiently, a certain amount of carbohydrate must be oxidized at the same time. Otherwise, more fat is broken down to
provide energy, and intermediate breakdown products appear in
excess. These are *ketones*, of which acetone and aceto-acetic acid
are examples. There are two important conditions in which insufficient carbohydrate is utilized to keep fat metabolism normal;
these are *uncontrolled diabetes mellitus* and *carbohydrate starvation*. In both, ketones appear in the urine.

   In patients who cannot eat and must be fed intravenously, fat can
be infused. A few fats are 'essential' in the sense that they are
needed in the body and cannot be made there, but significant
deficiency of essential fats takes many weeks to appear on a fat-free
diet. In patients who must be fed intravenously, temporary fat
deprivation is unimportant as long as sufficient carbohydrate can be
given to provide minimal caloric requirements. An intravenous fat
preparation can satisfy long-term needs (p. 185).

Protein

The building-blocks of protein are *amino-acids*, of which 22 are
known to be components of various proteins. Ten of these cannot be
made in the human body and must be supplied in the diet (essential
amino-acids); the other 12 can be made from available substances.
Amino-acids all contain carbon, hydrogen, oxygen and nitrogen in
their molecules, and are the chief nitrogen-containing substances in
the body.

   When protein is eaten, it is first broken down into amino-acids in
the gut. These are absorbed, and are then assembled into the
various proteins needed by the body. Each species of animal has its

own characteristic types of protein. Protein is present as an essential part of the structure of all cells and is most plentiful in muscle. It also circulates as plasma protein, which affects the distribution of water in the body (p. 10) and carries antibodies (in the gammaglobulins).

Body protein is continuously being broken down and replaced, and this occurs much more rapidly in starvation when carbohydrate and fat are not adequate for energy production.

All protein is eventually broken down into carbon dioxide and water (from carbon and hydrogen) and urea (from nitrogen). The latter is excreted in the urine (p. 91). The daily urinary nitrogen content (mostly as urea) gives a measure of the rate of protein breakdown.

It will be clear that while carbohydrate and fat are, to some extent, interchangeable (since their main function is to provide energy), the body must have a reliable supply of protein. The daily requirement is about 1 g per kg for an adult and 2 to 2·5 per kg for a child, while for each gram of nitrogen there should be available 200 non-protein Cal (837 kJ). 100 g of protein contain 18 g of nitrogen and should therefore be accompanied by 3600 non-protein Cal (15 062 kJ). Long-continued intravenous feeding soon leads to wasting unless protein can be supplied in some way. If tube-feeding is impossible, amino-acid solutions are available for intravenous use (p. 184).

The metabolic response to starvation

In a 24-hr period of starvation approximately 75 g of muscle protein and 160 g of adipose tissue fats are burned. About 180 g of glucose is produced from the liver glycogen and 145 g of this is used by the brain where it is completely metabolised. Other organs (heart, renal cortex, muscle) metabolise either fatty acids or ketones during starvation. The ketones are produced in the liver from fats and they can substitute for glucose as a source of energy for the brain which cannot utilize fats directly. These ketones thus help spare protein which would otherwise be converted to glucose once all the liver glycogen has been utilized.

The intravenous infusion of glucose into starving man leads to secretion of insulin which in turn inhibits protein brakdown in muscle. Administration of 100 g of glucose reduces the daily protein catabolism from 75 g to about 18 g.

The metabolic response to surgical operations

Certain metabolic disturbances are commonly observed in association with any operation, irrespective of its nature. The following causes have been identified:

1 Before and after most operations the patient is *starved of water and food* for several hours. In some patients food may have to be withheld for much longer.

2 *Endocrine adjustments* occur in response to any kind of trauma and therefore after a surgical operation. Whether these are beneficial or not is perhaps doubtful, but the practical point is that they occur. The more important adjustments are: (a) *Increased secretion of suprarenal steroids*, leading to protein breakdown, sodium retention and loss of potassium (p. 136). (b) *Increased secretion of thyroxine*, leading to an increase in metabolic rate. (c) *Increased secretion of antidiuretic hormone* (ADH), leading to retention of water (p. 12).

3 Should *infection* be present metabolic changes will be intensified.

4 Finally, *complications of the particular operation* may have metabolic effects. Renal failure, cardiac failure and loss of blood are examples.

As a result of the above, the following metabolic and associated changes are often seen.

1 *Oliguria* is caused by water restriction before operation and by increased secretion of ADH. The latter may be a direct result of trauma or secondary to sodium retention (p. 12). Oliguria may also be due to complicating renal failure.

2 *Retention of sodium* may be a normal response to sodium depletion but this is seldom present in cardiothoracic patients. In these, it is usually due to increased secretion of aldosterone (p. 12), renal failure (p. 96), and/or cardiac failure.

3 *Potassium depletion* has several possible causes. Prolonged cardiac failure before operation, especially if treated with diuretics, causes marked depletion. This is aggravated by increased cortisol secretion as a response to trauma. Hypoxia and acidosis complicating the postoperative period cause the cells to lose potassium. In general, the more extensive the operation the greater the postoperative potassium loss from the cells. The serum potassium concentration usually remains normal, but in the presence of renal failure it rises rapidly (p. 96).

4 *Breakdown of protein* is increased after operation, and is caused by increased cortisol secretion. The protein sparing effect of infused glucose does not occur after operation because insulin secretion and action is decreased by circulating steroids, adrenaline and thyroxine. Protein breakdown is demonstrated by finding an increased excretion of urea in the urine. Postoperative renal failure, in which excretion of urea is impaired (p. 96) therefore causes an unusually rapid increase in the blood urea concentration. Breakdown of the body proteins cannot be quickly repaired even if protein can be fed to the patient, because it takes time for the body to build up its proteins from absorbed amino-acids (p. 22).

5 *Loss of weight* is partly due to loss of protein but mainly to depletion of the fat stores (p. 20). Owing probably to thyroxine release, metabolic rate (p. 18) may double in the early postoperative period, and the extra energy comes mainly from fat.

6 *Pyrexia* occurs, even without infection, after most operations of any magnitude, and may last 2 or 3 days. It arises because extra heat is generated by increased metabolism faster than it can be dissipated (p. 27). Increased thyroxine secretion may be responsible.

Course of the metabolic response to cardiac operations

Both the severity and the duration of the metabolic response are related to the extent of the operation and its efficacy. The closure of a patent ductus arteriosus is an effective and relatively minor procedure and is usually followed by a mild response lasting only a couple of days. By the 3rd day such a patient would be apyrexial, retaining potassium, building protein, excreting a normal amount of urea, and eating a light diet. The patient who has had two or three valves replaced is older, has had cardiac failure before operation, has needed cardiopulmonary bypass during operation, may need IPPV (p. 250) for a day or two after operation and often has a low cardiac output for two or three days. He has a prolonged and severe metabolic response, lasting commonly up to a week and occasionally for several weeks.

Between these two extremes intermediate responses occur, and the postoperative metabolic management must take early account of the course which is likely to be followed. In the most simple of cases the supply of adequate intravenous water and calories (as 5 per cent glucose solution) for 24 hours is all that is necessary. Cases of intermediate severity will need potassium supplements and intravenous water and glucose (less often sodium) for 2 to 3 days. In the more severe cases there is no alternative but to carry out careful balance measurements (p. 13) of water, sodium and potassium and to judge infusion from these. Such patients lose fat and protein but provided there is an early prospect of their being able to eat it is not usual to do anything about this. It must be emphasized that the proper treatment of ventilatory failure, low cardiac output, pulmonary oedema and arrhythmias goes far to minimize the metabolic response in this difficult group of patients.

When catabolism is prolonged or eating is further delayed, oral or *total parenteral nutrition* may be necessary. This aims to provide by artificial means an adequate protein intake, a greater-than-normal caloric intake (from protein, carbohydrate and fat), and electrolytes, vitamins and other essential substances—all contained within the daily water requirement. It is more fully discussed on p. 185.

The regulation of body temperature

The temperature of the body is the net result of a balance between the rate of production and the rate of loss of heat. If production and loss of heat get out of balance, body temperature will rise or fall according to whether heat production or heat loss predominates.

Heat production is influenced by the following factors:
1 *The basal metabolic rate* (p. 18). This is regulated largely by the secretion of thyroid hormone. In the ICU, extra thyroxine secretion is part of the response to stress (p. 24) and basal metabolic rate (and thus heat production) increase in the postoperative period.
2 *Muscular activity.* 40 per cent of the energy developed by muscle during exercise is converted to useful mechanical work. The rest appears as heat. The muscles can thus produce a lot of heat, and shivering is a very important defence against a cold environment. When hypothermia has to be induced it is necessary to abolish shivering.

Heat loss is affected by many influences:
1 *The skin* acts as a radiator of heat. When its blood flow is high,

heat brought from the deeper tissues is lost to the environment. When skin blood-flow is reduced, skin temperature falls and radiation of heat diminishes.

2 *Evaporation of sweat* is another important way in which heat is lost; people sweat more on a hot day. In hyperpyrexia evaporative heat loss may be augmented by covering the patient with wet sheets upon which the draught from electric fans is directed.

3 The *warming and humidification of inspired air* in the respiratory deadspace (p. 75) means that heat is lost from the body. Expired gas is hotter and more humid than inspired gas. Panting is very important for dogs, who cannot sweat. In man, also, ventilation increases when body temperature is high.

Control of heat production and heat loss

In the hypothalamus, at the base of the brain, lies a *temperature-regulating centre*, which is sensitive to the temperature of the blood flowing through it. It also receives nerve impulses which convey information about skin temperature. From this 'evidence' of body temperature the centre 'decides' whether adjustments are necessary. These adjustments are made, over short periods, mainly by altering heat loss; skin circulation and the activity of sweat glands are increased or reduced according to whether the body is too warm or too cold. It must not be forgotten that in ordinary life conscious acts, like lighting fires, opening windows, putting on extra clothing and so on, play a most important part in the regulation of body temperature; these affect entirely heat loss. We also deliberately move about if we are cold; this is a conscious act involving heat production. At the unconscious level shivering is the short-term means of generating heat, and is brought about reflexly via the temperature-regulating centre. Note that the body has no way of *reducing* heat production below basal levels. Long exposure to a cold environment leads to a sustained increase in thyroxin secretion; this is brought about by the temperature-regulating centre via the pituitary gland.

Clinical aspects of temperature regulation

Infants have a poorly developed ability to regulate body temperature and readily lose heat if subjected even to normal room temperatures without clothes (p. 272). Even an adult who cannot move about is at a great disadvantage if uncovered, but because of a well-developed capacity for shivering and vasoconstriction can fend for himself much better than a baby. A baby's problem is largely its high surface area compared with weight; 'the heat-losing organ' is relatively big and the heat-generating tissues relatively small. This is one reason why a baby's metabolic rate has to be much higher than an adult's in relation to weight.

An adult's heat regulation may be upset by hypothalamic disease, as after head injury or cerebral air embolism, and hyperpyrexia may occur in these conditions. The pyrexia of the early postoperative period is probably due to thyroxine release. Infection causes pyrexia by an action on the heat-regulating centre.

2 The Autonomic Nervous System

Just as the muscles of the limbs and trunk are supplied with motor nerves, and the skin, joints and other structures with sensory nerves, so the internal organs have their own motor and sensory supply. This is called the *autonomic nervous system*, since it functions almost wholly free from conscious control. It regulates the activity of the heart and blood vessels, metabolism, body temperature, digestion and the secretion of many glands.

Anatomy

The autonomic nervous system comprises two distinct anatomical components which differ in function.

The sympathetic nervous system (Fig. 3). Impulses pass from a centre in the brain to the thoracic region of the spinal cord, where the sympathetic motor nerve cells lie. These cells transmit the impulses along their *preganglionic nerve fibres* to a second relay station, called a *ganglion*, outside the cord. From here, impulses travel along *postganglionic fibres* to the thoracic and abdominal organs, the blood vessels and other tissues.

Most of the sympathetic ganglia lie in pairs, one on each side of the spine. A bundle of connecting nerve fibres, extending from the base of the skull to the coccyx on each side, joins the ganglia together; it is the *sympathetic chain*, and it supplies the various regions as follows: head and neck (cervical ganglia), arms (stellate ganglia), heart and lungs (thoracic ganglia), legs (lumbar ganglia). Some ganglia lie outside the chain, e.g. the midline coeliac ganglion which supplies the abdominal viscera. The suprarenal medulla is a specialized sympathetic ganglion and receives preganglionic fibres; when these are stimulated, adrenaline and noradrenaline are released into the blood.

29

The parasympathetic nervous system (Fig. 3). Parasympathetic
ganglia lie mostly in the organs innervated. Preganglionic fibres
reach them through the 3rd, 7th, 9th and 10th cranial nerves and
convey impulses to the eye, the salivary glands, heart, lungs and
alimentary tract. This is the *'cranial outflow'*. A *'sacral outflow'*
travels in the sacral nerves and supplies the pelvic organs.

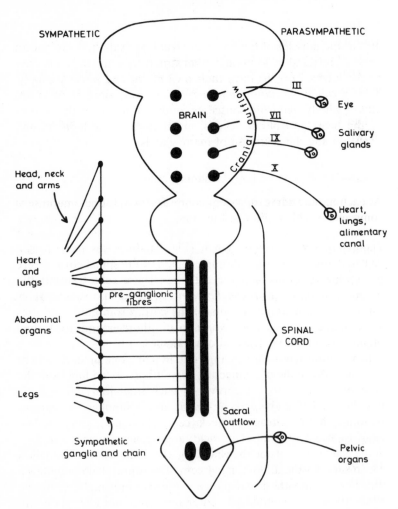

Fig. 3   Anatomy of the autonomic nervous system.

Autonomic sensory nerves. Autonomic reflexes must have a sensory component and visceral sensation is carried to the central nervous system by separate nerve fibres. Visceral sensory impulses do not usually reach consciousness but may do so, giving rise to angina pectoris, renal and bladder pain, and intestinal colic.

Physiology

1 *The sympathetic nervous system* is concerned with protection against external threats; it prepares the body for fight or flight, and helps to protect against haemmorrhage and cold.

2 *The parasympathetic nervous system* serves the 'domestic' affairs of the body, such as secretion of glands, storage of fuels and evacuation of bowels and bladder.

The effects of stimulation of the autonomic nervous system are shown in Table 5.

Transmission of nerve impulses in the autonomic nervous system

At each nerve ending, in ganglion or effector organ, the impulse is conveyed by the release of a chemical substance called a *transmitter*.

1 All preganglionic fibres (including those to the suprarenal glands) are *cholinergic,* that is their endings release *acetylcholine* (ACh).

2 All parasympathetic postganglionic fibres are also cholinergic.

3 As a general rule, sympathetic postganglionic fibre endings release *noradrenaline*, and are said to be *adrenergic*.

4 Sympathetic postganglionic fibres to the sweat glands and dilator fibres to vessels in muscle (Table 5) are the exception to rule **3,** in that their endings are *cholinergic*.

Drugs and the autonomic nervous system

Certain drugs mimic, and others block, the effects of autonomic stimulation (Table 5).

1 *Drugs which mimic sympathetic action (sympathomimetic drugs).* Certain drugs produce effects similar to those which result from stimulation of the sympathetic nervous system. It is evident from Table 5 that sympathetic stimulation results in widespread

Table 5   Effects of autonomic stimulation.

Organ	Sympathetic stimulation	Parasympathetic stimulation
Heart	Increase in force, rate, conduction and excitability	Decrease in force, rate, conduction and excitability
Lungs	Bronchi dilate	Bronchi constrict Secretions increase
Gut	Peristalsis inhibited Sphincters contract	Peristalsis increased Sphincters relax
Bladder	Wall relaxes Sphincter contracts	Wall contracts Sphincter relaxes
Arterioles: 1 Skin, mucosae 2 Muscle 3 Viscera 4 Lung	Constriction Mainly dilatation Constriction Constriction (weak)	Weak dilatation of doubtful physiological importance
Veins	Constriction	—
Eye	Pupil dilates	Pupil constricts
Salivary glands	Thick, viscid secretion	Profuse, watery secretion
Metabolic	Increased blood levels of glucose, insulin, and free fatty acids	—

changes but most sympathomimetic drugs produce only some of these. For example, one drug may stimulate the heart but have little effect on the peripheral vascular resistance, whereas another drug with a similar effect on the heart may sharply increase peripheral vascular resistance. To explain the differences in actions between these drugs it has been postulated that there are two types of *receptor* in the end organs affected by these drugs (e.g. in the arterioles, bronchi or myocardium).

Stimulation of the alpha (α) receptors results in constriction of arterioles and veins. Stimulation of the beta (β) receptors results in an increase in heart rate, improved conduction of the excitation wave and an increase in contractility. It also causes relaxation of arterioles in

Table 6 Sympathomimetic, parasympathomimetic and related blocking drugs.

	Stimulation of receptors		
	Alpha	Beta	Source
Sympathomimetic drugs			
Adrenaline (epinephrine)	+	+++	Suprarenal medulla
Noradrenaline (norepinephrine, levarterenol)	+++	++ (heart and bronchi only)	Suprarenal medulla and sympathetic endings
Dopamine	+	++	Noradrenaline precursor
Isoprenaline (isoproterenol)	−	+++	⎫
Dobutamine	+	++	⎪
Metaraminol	~ ++	+	⎪
Ephedrine	+	+	⎬ Do not occur naturally in the
Amphetamine	+	+	⎪ body
Fenoterol	−	++	⎪
Terbutaline	−	++	⎪
Salbutamol	−	++	⎪
Phenylephrine	++	−	⎭

Sympathetic blocking drugs	Receptor blocked	Comment
Phenoxybenzamine	Alpha	⎫
Phentolamine	Alpha	⎬ Have other actions
Tolazoline	Alpha	⎭
Propranolol	Beta	
Alprenolol	Beta	
Oxprenolol	Beta	
Pindolol	Beta	
Acebutolol	Beta	⎫
Atenolol	Beta	⎬ Cardioselective
Petoprolol	Beta	⎭

Parasympathomimetic drugs

Acetylcholine	(the physiological 'transmitter')
Carbachol	(a synthetic acetylcholine-like drug)
Neostigmine	(An anticholinesterase)
Edrophonium	(a short-acting anticholinesterase)

Acetylcholine (ACh) antagonists

Atropine	Blocks ACh action at parasympathetic postganglionic endings
Trimetaphan	Blocks ACh action in autonomic ganglia; therefore blocks transmission of sympathetic as well as parasympathetic impulses
Succinylcholine Tubocurarine	Block ACh action at motor end-plates in voluntary muscle. Two different mechanisms are involved (p. 37)

some regions, constriction of the veins and dilatation of bronchi.
Some drugs affect primarily the alpha receptors, some the beta
receptors, and some both. The main effects of commonly used drugs
are summarized in Table 6.

Some further refinement of this classification is helpful to allow
for the varying effects of drugs on beta receptors. Isoprenaline has a
powerful effect on all beta receptors and therefore produces a
tachycardia, improved conduction, increased contractility, together
with a reduction in systemic vascular resistance, venous constriction
and relaxation of bronchi. By contrast drugs such as fenoterol,
terbutaline and salbutamol have come into use because they dilate
bronchi but have very little cardiac effect. Beta receptors have
therefore been divided into two categories, beta 1 and beta 2.
Cardiac responses are due to stimulation of beta 1 receptors and
dilatation of bronchi and arterioles to stimulation of beta 2 receptors.

2 *Sympathetic blocking drugs* reduce or abolish the effects of
sympathetic stimulation and also block the actions of sympathomimetic substances. They affect alpha and beta receptors selec-
tively. Cardioselective beta receptor blocking drugs block the beta 1
receptors but have much less effect on beta 2 receptors; they are
therefore safer in patients with a wheeze where blockade of broncho-
dilatation (beta 2 receptors) can be very troublesome. They are also
safer in diabetic patients. Blockade of beta receptors accentuates
the risk of hypoglycaemia but this is much less worrisome when beta
2 receptors are not blocked.

3 *Parasympathetic substances* mimic parasympathetic action.
Acetylcholine is the one that occurs in the body and is the chemical
transmitter of nerve impulses:
a   In the central nervous system.
b   In autonomic ganglia, both sympathetic and parasympathetic.
c   At parasympathetic, postganglionic nerve endings.
d   At the sympathetic postganglionic nerve endings in sweat glands
and the blood vessels in muscle.
e   At the endings of motor nerves in voluntary muscle ('motor end
plates').

Very little is known about the action at site **a**. Site **e** does not
concern the parasympathetic system and is discussed later.

When ACh is released, either in a ganglion or at a parasympathetic postganglionic ending, it is quickly destroyed by an

enzyme called *cholinesterase*. A substance which prevents this destruction of ACh is called an anticholinesterase, and many such substances are known (Table 6). Anticholinesterases cause released ACh to persist, and therefore they magnify the effects of ACh; in other words they are parasympathomimetic.

4 *Parasympathetic blocking drugs* are ACh antagonists. They can be divided into (a) those that act at the autonomic ganglia—ganglion blocking drugs—and (b) those that act at the postganglionic nerve endings e.g. atropine.

The reader is advised not to try to learn the effects of administering all these drugs individually. Instead, from a knowledge of sympathetic and parasympathetic actions (Table 5), and of a particular drug's basic action (Table 6), its various effects can be deduced in considerable detail, and without risk of errors of memory. It remains only to mention the main uses of the more frequently used drugs.

Uses of autonomic drugs

Sympathomimetic drugs

Isoprenaline has a pure beta-stimulating effect. Adrenaline also has a strong beta-stimulating effect but also produces vasoconstriction in some regions. Although noradrenaline stimulates the heart it has a strong alpha-stimulating effect on the peripheral vessels and the resulting increase in systemic vascular resistance overshadows the cardiac effect. The action of metaraminol is similar and although less powerful than noradrenaline this drug has the advantage that it can be given intra-muscularly. Phenylephrine has a pure alpha-stimulating effect but does not cause appreciable stimulation of the heart.

Some years ago, drugs causing peripheral vasoconstriction were often used to raise the blood pressure in patients with shock. However, the blood flow to vital regions does not necessarily increase, despite the rise in blood pressure, and indeed some organs, especially the kidneys, receive less blood. The increase in blood pressure usually puts a greater load on the heart without producing the desired improvement in perfusion of vital regions. Vasoconstrictor drugs are therefore rarely used in shock nowadays. In acute circulatory collapse adrenaline is sometimes administered in the hope

that its combined effect on the heart and on the peripheral vascula-
ture may maintain a sufficient blood flow to the brain and heart to
carry the patient through a critical period.

Dopamine has some vasoconstricting effect but, in doses lower
than 10 μg per kg per min (probably lower still in babies) it dilates
renal arterioles. It has a potent inotropic action (p. 49) and will
sometimes increase cardiac output without the pronounced tachycardia caused by isoprenaline. It is also useful in patients with
frequent ventricular ectopic beats. Dobutamine does not have a
specific renal vasodilatory effect, but, at low doses, has a mild
general vasodilator effect. For practical purposes the effects of
dopamine and dobutamine can be considered very similar.

Sympathetic blocking drugs

The alpha receptor blocker prazosin is used to reduce systemic
vascular resistance in hypertension or chronic heart failure.
Phenoxybenzamine has been used to improve peripheral blood flow
in shock but, because of its prolonged action, has largely been
replaced by shorter acting vasodilating drugs (p. 118). Beta receptor blocking drugs are used to reduce the effects of sympathetic
impulses to the heart in the treatment and prevention of cardiac
arrhythmias. They are also effective in the treatment of angina,
largely by limiting fluctuations in cardiac work with stress and
exercise. Care is required in patients with poor myocardial function
where removal of autonomic tone may precipitate heart failure.

Parasympathomimetic drugs

Carbachol, a long-acting form of ACh, is sometimes given to relieve
postoperative urinary retention. Neostigmine (an anticholinesterase, Table 6) is extensively used to reverse the action of
muscle-relaxants (p. 38) and in the treatment of myasthenia
gravis. Its side-effects, in big doses, include colic, salivation, bradycardia and bronchoconstriction, and these may be prevented by
atropine. Atropine does *not* block the action of neostigmine on
voluntary muscle. An excess of neostigmine causes widespread
muscular twitching and weakness. It is important to distinguish this
from the weakness due to myasthenia or relaxant drug, for which
the neostigmine has been given. Neostigmine inactivates cholinesterase temporarily. Prolonged or permanent inactivation (leading

to the patient's death) may result from exposure to 'organo-phosphorus' insecticides; treatment demands artificial respiration, atropine and a 'cholinesterase reactivator'.

Parasympathetic antagonists

Atropine is used (a) to increase heart rate and cardiac output when these are reduced by vagal overactivity, (b) to diminish salivary and bronchial secretions, e.g. during anaesthesia, and (c) to block un-wanted side effects of neostigmine (see above). Atropine dilates the pupils (Table 5), and if atropine has been given the pupils are no longer a reliable guide to the presence of cerebral damage after cardiac arrest.

Atropine abolishes sweating (sympathetic ACh activity (p. 31) and this may cause hyperpyrexia especially in febrile children. Large or repeated doses of atropine may block ACh transmission in the central nervous system causing restlessness, irritability, dis-orientation, hallucinations and delirium.

Drugs affecting neuromuscular transmission

When a nerve impulse reaches the motor end plate in a voluntary muscle, a little 'packet' of ACh molecules is released. The ACh acts on a 'receptor' on the muscle fibre and muscle contraction is initiated. Released ACh is normally destroyed very quickly by cholinesterase. Strong muscle contractions are achieved by impulses being sent down more nerve fibres, or more frequently down the same nerve fibres, thus releasing more ACh. Drugs that block the action of ACh on the muscle fibres stop contraction by preventing the nerve impulses from being transmitted to the mus-cle. These drugs are called muscle relaxants.

1 *Tubocurarine, alcuronium and pancuronium* compete with ACh for receptor sites. The more drug present, the fewer receptor sites remain available for ACh and the greater the degree of paralysis. All voluntary muscles are rapidly paralysed by an intravenous dose of these muscle relaxants and the effect lasts for about 1 hr, depend-ing on the size of the dose. Paralysis of the respiratory muscles makes artificial ventilation essential. Muscle relaxants do not cause unconsciousness and a paralysed, ventilated patient remains awake unless a hypnotic drug is also given. Tubocurarine and alcuronium

have some blocking action in autonomic ganglia and blood pressure falls transiently when they are given. Both these drugs may also release histamine which can cause hypotension, urticaria and bronchoconstriction in sensitive patients. Pancuronium does not have these side effects.

These *competitive inhibitors* of ACh can be displaced from the receptor sites by increasing the local concentration of ACh. The administration of an anticholinesterase such as neostigmine, which prevents the destruction of released ACh, thus reverses the muscle paralysis.

2 *Succinylcholine* acts differently; it is not a competitive inhibitor of ACh, but renders the muscle fibre insensitive to the action of ACh. This effect is short lived (less than 5 minutes) because the succinylcholine is rapidly destroyed by cholinesterase. Because the muscle fibre is insensitive to ACh, administration of neostigmine will not reverse the action of succinylcholine but may well prolong the paralysis by inhibiting cholinesterase.

Muscle relaxants are administered almost routinely during major surgical operations, because they allow much smaller non-toxic doses of anaesthetic drugs to be used. They may also be used in the treatment of convulsions, for example status epilepticus and tetanus. Some respiratory units use muscle relaxants to facilitate the control of artificial ventilation.

3 The Heart and Circulation

The cardiovascular system serves three main functions.

1 Oxygen and nutrient materials are carried to all body tissues to maintain their nutrition and metabolic function.

2 The blood is then carried to the lungs which discharge the carbon dioxide produced by metabolism and replace the oxygen used by the tissues.

3 Other waste products of metabolism, and many drugs, are carried to the appropriate organs for breakdown and elimination. Some are carried to the kidneys and excreted in the urine. Others are carried to the liver, broken down, and either excreted into the bile and discharged in the faeces, or returned in altered form to the blood to be transported to the kidneys.

The heart pumps blood through the arteries, capillaries and veins which make up the peripheral circulation. At rest it has to pump at only a modest rate but during exercise its output must increase sharply. The peripheral circulation must be adaptable so that blood can be distributed where it is needed most—for instance, during exercise, blood flow to muscles must be greatly increased. Abnormal situations, e.g. haemorrhage, make special demands both on the heart and on the peripheral circulation. To tide a patient over his crucial stay in the ICU demands a basic understanding of the structure and function of the heart and peripheral circulation and of the way in which each responds to stress.

Anatomy of the heart

Only basic anatomy, relevant to normal and abnormal function, is reviewed here.

The heart consists of four chambers, right and left atria and right and left ventricles (Fig. 4). The right atrium receives venous blood from the superior and inferior venae cavae and conveys it through the tricuspid valve to the right ventricle. When the right ventricle contracts it pumps blood through the pulmonary valve to the pulmonary artery. The tricuspid valve has three leaflets whose free edges are held in place by cords (the chordae tendineae) which are attached to the ventricular wall by papillary muscles. The pulmonary valve consists of three cusps built in such a way that they support themselves and do not require chordae tendineae.

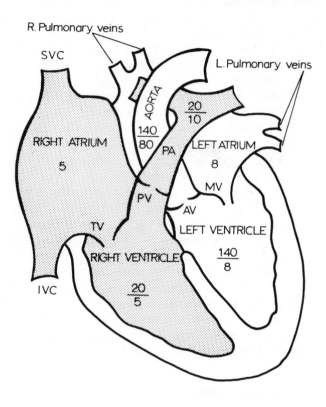

Fig. 4 Anatomy of the heart. The right side of the heart is shaded. SVC, superior vena cava; IVC, inferior vena cava; PA, main pulmonary artery; TV, tricuspid valve; PV, pulmonary valve; MV, mitral valve; AV, aortic valve. Typical pressures are shown. Atrial pressures are the mean for the cardiac cycle.

The left atrium receives blood from the pulmonary veins and pumps it through the mitral valve into the left ventricle. When the left ventricle contracts, it pumps blood through the aortic valve into the aorta. The mitral valve has two cusps whose free edges are held in place by chordae tendineae while the aortic valve, like the pulmonary, has three self-supporting cusps. The mitral and tricuspid valves are called the atrioventricular valves (A-V valves) because they separate the atria from the ventricles while the aortic and pulmonary valves are called semilunar valves because their cusps resemble half-moons.

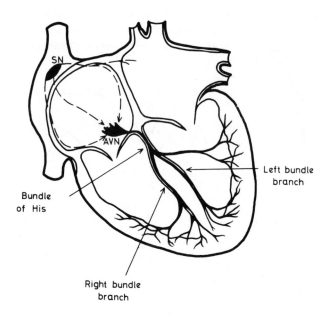

Fig. 5 Conducting tissue of the heart. SN, sinus node; AVN, atrioventricular node.

The conducting tissue of the heart

Each heart beat is triggered by an electrical impulse (called the *excitation wave*) which passes through the heart along a pathway of specialized conducting tissue (Fig. 5). This impulse normally starts in a small group of specialized cells situated near the junction of the superior vena cava and right atrium and called the *sinus node*. In

other words, the sinus node is the normal *pacemaker* of the heart.
From here the excitation wave passes through the muscle of both
atria to the *atrioventricular node* (the A-V node) in the right atrial
wall just above the interventricular septum. It enters this septum
through the *A-V bundle*, otherwise known as the *bundle of His*,
which then divides into the right and left bundles. After traversing
these bundles the impulse spreads through the Purkinje fibres to the
muscle of the right and left ventricles.

Blood supply of the heart

Like all tissues the heart muscle has its own blood supply. The
arteries are the coronary arteries which are described in the section
on ischaemic heart disease (p. 220). The major coronary arteries

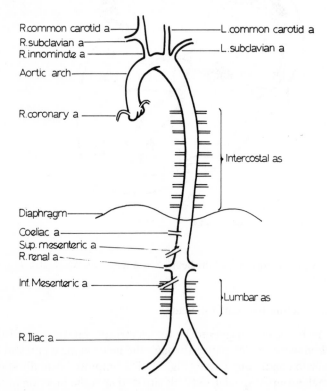

Fig. 6   Main branches of the aorta.

run on the epicardial surface of the heart and the small arteries directly supplying the myocardium pass from the epicardial to the endocardial region. Where the blood supply is limited by ischaemia or where the oxygen demand is excessive, as for example in the hypertrophied heart of the patient with severe aortic stenosis, the subendocardial region is especially vulnerable.

Anatomy of the peripheral circulation

The aorta gives off arteries to each major area of the body (Fig. 6). The two coronary arteries, right and left, arise just above the aortic valve. The subclavian arteries to the arms, and the carotid arteries to the head and neck, arise from the arch of the aorta as it curves backwards to to pass down the chest and through the diaphragm. In the abdomen arise the coeliac artery which supplies organs in the upper abdomen, the superior mesenteric artery passing to the small bowel, the renal arteries which supply the kidneys and the inferior mesenteric artery which passes to the large bowel. The aorta ends by dividing into right and left iliac arteries which supply the femoral arteries to the legs.

These main arteries in turn divide like the branches of a tree into arteries of progressively diminishing size (Fig. 7). The smallest arteries feed the arterioles which lead to an extensive network of tiny vessels, the capillaries. The capillaries drain into venules which unite to form small veins. As more small veins unite, larger veins are formed and eventually the largest branches drain into either the superior or the inferior vena cava. This whole vascular bed is called the *peripheral* or *systemic circulation*.

The portal circulation is a specialized part of the systemic circulation. It consists of the venous drainage of the spleen and most of the alimentary tract, which passes via the portal vein to a second set of capillaries in the liver. From these, blood is collected in the hepatic veins which join the inferior vena cava.

The pulmonary arteries branch repeatedly until the pulmonary arterioles are reached. These feed the pulmonary capillaries which unite to form pulmonary venules and larger pulmonary veins, and eventually four main pulmonary veins (two from each lung) enter the left atrium. The vascular bed within the lungs is called the *pulmonary circulation*.

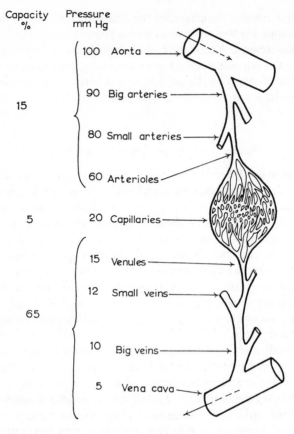

Capacity %	Pressure mm Hg	
	100	Aorta
15	90	Big arteries
	80	Small arteries
	60	Arterioles
5	20	Capillaries
	15	Venules
	12	Small veins
65	10	Big veins
	5	Vena cava

Fig. 7 Diagram to show components of the systemic vascular bed. The percentage of the total blood volume in each segment is shown in the column headed 'capacity'. The missing 15 per cent is contained in the pulmonary vascular bed and heart.

The pressure in the aorta must be high enough to drive blood through the arteries, arterioles and capillaries into veins, and thence to the right atrium. The aorta must be stoutly built to withstand this pressure and its walls therefore have strong elastic fibres as well as a thick muscular coat. As the blood passes through the vascular bed, pressure gradually falls and in the smaller arteries the walls are therefore not so thick. The arterioles have only a muscular coat and in the capillaries even this is lost. The capillaries are tiny vessels lined only by a single layer of cells and form a very extensive network reaching virtually every cell in the body. The veins, too are relatively thin-walled although all but the smallest contain some elastic fibres and a thin muscular coat. At intervals along the length of the larger veins there are valves which permit flow only towards the heart; these can easily be demonstrated in your own arm.

Function of the heart

The heart consists mainly of a special type of muscle which is unique in that it contracts spontaneously and rhythmically throughout life. It fills and empties in a regular and systematic fashion which will now be described.

The cardiac cycle

For each heartbeat there is a period when the ventricles contract to eject blood (*systole*) and a period when the ventricles relax to permit refilling (*diastole*). These events occur almost simultaneously on both sides of the heart and the period including one systole and the following diastole is called the *cardiac cycle*.

Electrical events of the cardiac cycle. (Fig. 22, p. 143) The beginning of the excitation wave in the sinus node is not recorded in the electrocardiogram (ECG or EKG) but the spread of the impulse through the atria produces the *P wave*. Passage of the impulse through the A-V node, bundle of His and right and left bundle branches produces no deflection in the ECG but is responsible for the slight delay between the P wave and the beginning of QRS. The *QRS complex* is produced by the spread of the excitation wave through the right and left ventricular muscle. The *T wave* is produced as the ventricles recover from the passage of the excitation wave.

It is the spread of the excitation wave which makes cardiac muscle contract. Thus the passage of the impulse through the atria (producing the P wave) makes the atria contract and its passage through the ventricles (producing the QRS complex) makes the ventricles contract.

Mechanical events of the cardiac cycle. Fig. 8, which depicts pressure changes in the left side of the heart, will repay careful and repeated study.

Towards the end of diastole, just after the P wave of the ECG, the left atrium contracts and accelerates the flow of blood through the open mitral valve into the left ventricle. The QRS complex then occurs and following this the ventricle contracts. The pressure in the ventricle very soon rises above that in the atrium and the mitral valve closes, preventing blood from flowing backwards from the ventricle to the atrium. Closure of the mitral valve produces the first heart sound (S1). The ventricular pressure continues to rise rapidly

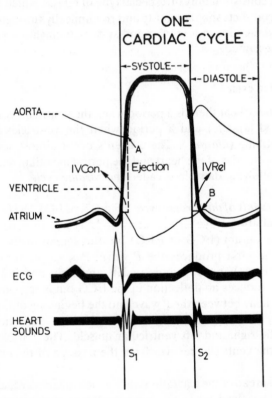

Fig. 8 Events of the cardiac cycle, showing pressures in the aorta, left ventricle and left atrium, the ECG and the heart sounds. S_1, first heart sound; S_2, second heart sound; IVCon, isovolumic contraction; IVRel, isovolumic relaxation (see also Fig. 22, p. 143).

and soon exceeds that in the aorta, forcing the aortic valve to open (point A). Blood is then ejected into the aorta until, as the ventricle relaxes, the ventricular pressure falls below that in the aorta. This causes the aortic valve to close, preventing reflux of blood from the aorta to the ventricle and producing the second heart sound (S2). Pressure in the ventricle drops rapidly until it falls below that in the atrium; at this point (B) the mitral valve reopens and blood again moves freely from the atrium to the ventricle.

During the whole cardiac cycle, blood is returning from the pulmonary veins to the left atrium. It can pass from the atrium to the ventricle only when the mitral valve is open, and this is during diastole. On the other hand blood is ejected from the ventricle to the aorta only during systole. In other words, ventricular filling takes place during diastole while ventricular ejection takes place during systole. Note that systole has three components; *isovolumic contraction* when the pressure is rising but, because both mitral and aortic valves are closed, ventricular volume does not change; *ejection* between opening and closure of the aortic valve; and *isovolumic relaxation* from aortic valve closure to mitral valve reopening. If aortic pressure is stable the following ratio gives a measure of ventricular contractility.

$$\frac{\text{isovolumic contraction time}}{\text{ejection time}}$$

If myocardial function is impaired the rate of contraction is slowed and the ratio increases.

Events on the right side of the heart occur almost simultaneously with those on the left. Thus the tricuspid valve opens and closes about the same time as the mitral valve and the pulmonary valve opens and closes about the same time as the aortic valve.

Pressures in the heart. The pressures in the systemic circuit (as recorded in routine blood pressure measurements) are higher than those in the pulmonary circuit. Representative pressures are shown in Fig. 4. Systemic pressure is much lower in early than in later life; arterial pressure is usually about 70/50 mmHg in the newborn infant, rising to about 90/60 in the toddler, 100/70 in the older child and 120/80 in the teenager. The difference between systolic and diastolic pressures is the *pulse pressure*; if the arterial pressure is 140/80, the pulse pressure is 60 mmHg.

The control of cardiac output

The volume of blood pumped by the heart each minute is called the *cardiac output*. The volume ejected during each systole is called the *stroke volume*. An average adult's resting stroke volume is about 70 ml. If the heart rate is 80 the cardiac output is (70×80) ml = 5600 ml per min or 5·6 l per min. Thus:

$$\text{Cardiac output} = \text{heart rate} \times \text{stroke volume}$$

To increase the cardiac output, for instance with exercise, the heart rate or the stroke volume, or both, must increase.

The heart rate. The heart is slowed by stimulation of the *vagus nerve* (X, Fig. 3, p. 30). Impulses pass continuously down the vagus nerve; anything which blocks vagal action will thus increase the heart rate. The vagus nerve slows the heart by releasing *acetylcholine* whose effect is blocked by the administration of atropine (p. 37).

An increase in heart rate also results from stimulation of the *cardiac sympathetic nerves*. These nerves stimulate the pacemaker cells by releasing noradrenaline. Circulating adrenaline, released from the adrenal gland, and noradrenaline increase the heart rate in the same way, but the effect of the sympathetic nerves is more important under normal circumstances.

The stroke volume. Stroke volume may be increased in two ways: (1) by increasing the filling of the heart, and (2) by increasing the efficiency of contraction.

1 Increased filling of the heart. Within certain limits, cardiac muscle fibres contract more forcibly the more they are stretched before contraction begins. This is called *Starling's Law* of the heart. Stretching of the fibres is achieved by increasing venous return to the heart, which results in greater filling. The more forceful contraction which ensues empties the heart more effectively, thus increasing the stroke volume. A healthy ventricle will eject something like two thirds of its volume with each systole. This can be assessed at cineangiography, where the *ejection fraction*, that is the ratio:

$$\frac{\text{stroke volume}}{\text{end-diastolic volume}}$$

is frequently measured. For example a stroke volume of 70 ml and an end-diastolic volume of 110 ml gives an ejection fraction of:

$$\frac{70}{110} = 0.64.$$

An ejection fraction below 0·5 is abnormal and an ejection fraction of 0·25 indicates a critical impairment of left ventricular function. The Starling mechanism is important in maintaining an equal output of the right and left ventricles. It is obvious that the two sides of the heart must pump blood at the same rate. For instance, if the right side were to pump more than the left, blood would quickly accumulate in the lungs causing pulmonary congestion and reducing the volume in the systemic circuit.

2 Improved efficiency of contraction. In addition to increasing the heart rate (called the *chronotropic* effect) the cardiac sympathetic nerves and circulating adrenaline have a direct *inotropic* effect on cardiac muscle, i.e. they increase both the *speed and the strength of contraction.*

These three mechanisms—increased heart rate, increased filling of the heart and increased efficiency of contraction—normally operate together to increase the cardiac output as required.

Function of the peripheral circulation

The peripheral circulation must (1) distribute the cardiac output so that each region of the body receives an adequate blood-flow; (2) perfuse the tissues so that the nutrition of all cells is maintained; and (3) return blood to the heart fast enough to maintain the cardiac output. There are essentially three parts of the circulation, each concerned with one of these functions.

1 The arterial bed (including the arterioles) maintains an adequate blood pressure for perfusion and it distributes the cardiac output around the body according to needs.

2 The capillary bed brings the blood into close relationship with all body cells.

3 The veins return blood to the heart at the rate required to maintain cardiac output.

Function of the arterial bed

The pressure within the arteries gradually falls as blood flows towards the periphery because the blood vessels offer resistance to flow. It obviously requires more pressure to push fluid through a narrow than through a wide tube, and if fluid flows at the same rate through two tubes of equal length the pressure will drop more along a narrow tube than along a wider one. We can thus define the resistance of a tube in terms of flow and pressure, and we can define vascular resistance in the same way.

$$\text{Systemic vascular resistance} = \frac{\text{pressure drop along the systemic vascular bed}}{\text{rate of flow through the systemic vascular bed}}$$

$$= \frac{\text{(Aortic—right atrial) mean pressure in mmHg*}}{\text{Cardiac output in 1 per min}}$$

which, using typical figures

$$= \frac{100-5}{5\cdot6} \text{ 'Resistance units'}$$

or about 15 'Resistance units'

$$\text{Pulmonary vascular resistance} = \frac{\text{(Pulmonary arterial – left atrial) mean pressure in mmHg}}{\text{Cardiac output in 1 per min}} = \frac{15-10}{5\cdot6}$$

or about 1 'Resistance unit'.

*Because the right atrial pressure is very small compared with aortic pressure, this equation approximates to:

$$\text{Resistance} = \frac{\text{aortic pressure}}{\text{cardiac output}}$$

In turn, this can be rewritten:

$$\text{Aortic pressure} = \text{cardiac output} \times \text{resistance}$$

Because the resistance to flow through the pulmonary vascular bed is much lower, pressures in the pulmonary circuit are lower than systemic.

There is a much greater drop in pressure along the arteries than along the capillaries and veins. This is because the arteries offer greater resistance to flow than do the capillaries or veins. Most of the pressure drop occurs in the small arteries and arterioles because these are the vessels which offer the greatest resistance to flow. They are therefore sometimes called the *resistance vessels*. As we shall see, vascular resistance varies continuously in order to maintain a relatively constant arterial pressure during fluctuations in cardiac output. Furthermore the resistance may change in one region more than in another so that blood can be directed where it is needed most. Flow to regions with a high resistance is reduced, and flow to other regions is increased.

Regional blood flow. The approximate distribution of cardiac output at rest is shown in Table 7.

Table 7   Distribution of cardiac output at rest.

Region	Cardiac output received (%)
Brain	15
Heart (coronary flow)	5
Kidney	20
Bowel	10
Muscle	20
Skin	10
Other regions	20

Function of the capillary bed

Because the wall of the capillary is a single layer of flattened cells, oxygen, carbon dioxide and other metabolites can pass easily across it. Exchange of these substances takes place between the interstitial fluid and cells, and cellular metabolism is maintained. Under resting conditions only part of each regional capillary bed is perfused with blood at any given moment. Capillaries in one area will be perfused for a time, close down for a short period, and reopen later. This shifting, intermittent flow is adequate to maintain the nutrition of the cells and it avoids pooling of blood in the capillaries which would occur if the whole bed were open at once.

Function of the veins

The importance of the venous bed lies in its large *capacity*, which can be adjusted by venous constriction to meet varying needs. The veins (and for this purpose we include the portal circulation) usually contain about two thirds of the total blood-volume, that is about

3300 ml. Because of their large capacity the veins are sometimes referred to as the *capacitance vessels*. In effect the veins act as a store of blood, returning it to the heart as required to maintain the cardiac output.

Control of the peripheral circulation

Control of the arterial bed

Three main factors affect the arteries and arterioles: (1) the sympathetic nervous system, (2) circulating substances such as adrenaline, and (3) local effects.

1   Stimulation of the sympathetic nervous system releases noradrenaline at nerve endings and produces constriction of the small arteries and arterioles (the resistance vessels), thus raising the peripheral vascular resistance. Some tissues have more sympathetic nerves than others. Stimulation of the sympathetic nerves therefore increases resistance and decreases flow in these regions more than in others. The resistance vessels in the kidney, skin, spleen and mesenteric vessels have a richer sympathetic nerve supply than those in muscle, and resistance vessels in the heart and brain have a negligible sympathetic nerve supply. Stimulation of the sympathetic nerves therefore sharply reduces the blood flow to the kidneys, skin, spleen and bowel; produces a moderate drop in flow to muscle; and does not reduce the flow to the heart or brain at all.

Infusion of noradrenaline mimics the stimulation of sympathetic nerves; both stimulate the α-receptors (p. 32).

2   The release of adrenaline from the adrenal glands into the circulation has a double effect. There is some stimulation of alpha receptors, causing vasoconstriction, but in addition there is stimulation of a second group of receptors (β-receptors, p. 32) in the arterial walls. In those tissues containing beta receptors, the amount of vasoconstriction produced by the release of adrenaline is therefore much less than that produced by stimulation of the sympathetic nerves. These tissues include muscle, the bowel and the heart. Under ordinary circumstances stimulation of the sympathetic nerves is more important than release of adrenaline.

3   Local effects:

a   Temperature. Heat dilates arterioles both by a local action and indirectly through the heat-regulating centre in the brain (p. 27).

Vasodilatation in the skin is essential for the rapid dissipation of heat from the body.

b Carbon dioxide stimulates the sympathetic nerves *centrally*, causing a rise in resistance and a rise in blood pressure. When the P_{CO_2} becomes very high, this effect is overshadowed by the *local* action of CO_2 on the resistance vessels which causes them to dilate, and the blood pressure falls. Resistance vessels in the brain are very susceptible to this dilator action of CO_2, and are hardly affected by sympathetic stimulation (see above). Cerebral vasodilatation thus occurs even with a slight rise in tissue P_{CO_2}.

c Hypoxia, like excess of CO_2, stimulates the sympathetic nerves *centrally*, and thus constricts resistance vessels generally. *Locally*, if it becomes marked, it dilates the systemic resistance vessels by direct action. The resistance vessels in muscle are particularly susceptible to local hypoxia.

d Acidosis. The general release of acid in *metabolic acidosis* opposes sympathetic vasoconstriction in all tissues, causing a generalized dilatation of resistance vessels. A good deal of lactic acid is released in exercising muscle, where it completely over-rides the influence of the sympathetic nerves. In this way exercising muscles are assured of the lion's share of the cardiac output.

Under normal circumstances these three mechanisms act together to ensure that all regions receive an adequate blood-supply. Stimulation of the sympathetic nerves will raise the total resistance of the systemic circuit and the arterial blood-pressure. Blood flow to the kidneys, skin, spleen, bowel and muscle may be reduced but these tissues can easily withstand a period of reduced blood-flow. On the other hand the flow to the heart and brain is maintained to the last ditch. During exercise the local effect of lactic acid ensures that muscles receive a generous blood-flow.

Control of the capillary bed

Flow through the capillaries is controlled almost entirely by local factors. In tissues receiving a limited capillary–flow the P_{O_2} and pH fall while the P_{CO_2} rises. These changes dilate the arterioles leading to this part of the capillary bed, allowing blood to flow freely until P_{O_2}, pH and P_{CO_2} are restored to normal. The arterioles then narrow again and the cycle is repeated.

Control of the veins

Because it is more difficult to study changes in the veins than changes in arteries our knowledge of the control of veins is less complete. There are however three mechanisms which modify the volume or capacity of the venous bed and the rate at which venous blood is returned to the heart. These are:

The action of sympathetic nerves. Stimulation of the sympathetic nerves causes the veins throughout the body to constrict, or in other words to increase their tone. This reduces the capacity of the venous bed and raises the pressure within it. The presence of valves within the veins ensures that this constriction drives blood towards the heart.

Unlike the resistance vessels, the veins, or capacitance vessels, do not show variation in constriction from one region to another. Sympathetic stimulation thus produces generalized venous constriction.

Release of adrenaline from the adrenal glands. Adrenaline has the same effect on the veins as stimulation of the sympathetic nerves. Venous tone is increased, the capacity of the venous bed is reduced and there is increased venous return to the heart. Under ordinary circumstances this is much less important than sympathetic stimulation.

The 'muscle pump'. During exercise the veins within muscles are compressed each time the muscle contracts, and the presence of valves within the veins ensures that this produces an increased venous return to the heart.

Function of the pulmonary circulation

In a sense the task of the pulmonary circulation is much simpler than that of the systemic circulation. It merely has to perfuse the capillaries surrounding the alveoli to permit exchange of oxygen and carbon dioxide. The rather complex mechanisms which control the systemic circulation therefore play a smaller part in the control of the pulmonary circulation. As we have already seen, the resistance in the pulmonary circulation is much lower than in the systemic circulation, and the pressure in the arteries is therefore lower. In fact, in the upright position, there is barely enough pressure within the pulmonary arteries to keep the capillaries open near the apices of the lungs and the flow is therefore greater towards the bases. At rest there is little variation in the pulmonary vascular resistance from moment to moment.

As in systemic organs, the capillary bed is only partly perfused at any one time. The pulmonary veins are relatively short and they do not contain valves.

Control of the pulmonary circulation

In general the pulmonary resistance vessels passively transmit whatever flow they receive from the right heart. Opening up the unused parts of the arterial and capillary beds permits pulmonary flow to increase two- or three-fold with little increase in pulmonary arterial pressure. The pulmonary bed has considerable ability to alter its capacity, largely under the influence of the sympathetic nerves. The pulmonary vessels usually contain about 12–15 per cent of the total blood volume, and constriction of the pulmonary veins by sympathetic stimulation can reduce this significantly. Hypoxia constricts the pulmonary resistance vessels.

Overall control of the circulation

We have seen that vagal stimulation slows the heart, whereas sympathetic stimulation speeds the heart, increases contractility (and therefore stroke volume), constricts resistance vessels thereby raising the systemic vascular resistance and redistributing blood flow, and constricts veins thereby increasing the venous return to the heart and so helping to increase stroke volume. Overall control of sympathetic and vagal activity comes from the *vagal and sympathetic centres* in the brain. These centres are connected so that their effects are coordinated; for example, stimulation of the sympathetic centre combines with depression of the vagal centre to produce an increased heart rate. One part of the sympathetic centre is concerned more with producing a response in the peripheral circulation (the *vasomotor centre*) while another less well-defined region is concerned primarily with control of the heart (the *cardiac centre*).

In turn these centres receive afferent (that is, incoming) impulses from many regions of the body. For example, the *vagal centre* receives afferent impulses from the respiratory tract, gastrointestinal tract, heart, blood vessels and muscles. Intubation of the trachea or puncture of a brachial artery sometimes causes a dramatic fall in heart rate by stimulating the vagal centre.

Similarly, the *sympathetic centre* receives impulses from many regions of which three are most important:

High-pressure receptors. The wall of each common carotid artery, at the point where it branches into external and internal carotid arteries, contains special receptors which are sensitive to stretch. When arterial pressure is high, these receptors are stimulated and send impulses to the sympathetic and vagal centres. The receptor areas are called the *carotid sinuses.* They are the main arterial-pressure receptors but similar receptors are present elsewhere in the arterial system.

A rise in the mean arterial pressure or the pulse pressure increases the number of impulses reaching the brain from the carotid sinuses, and these *diminish the output of the vasomotor centre.* As a result, systemic vascular resistance is reduced and the rise in blood pressure is counteracted (remember that blood pressure = cardiac output × systemic vascular resistance; see note p. 50). A fall in blood pressure, on the other hand, diminishes the number of impulses from the carotid sinuses to the brain, and the opposite reflex occurs; *the output of the vasomotor centre is increased* and blood pressure rises. By means of these reflexes, called *baroreceptor reflexes*, the blood pressure is prevented from rising or falling beyond quite narrow limits. The mechanism is very important in maintaining blood pressure in the presence of cardiac failure or haemorrhage.

These reflex changes in blood pressure are usually accompanied by changes in heart rate due to simultaneous effects on the cardiac centre and the vagal centre. Thus a rise in blood pressure is minimized by the baroreceptor reflex and is accompanied by bradycardia, while a fall in blood pressure is minimized by the baroreceptor reflex and is accompanied by tachycardia.

Low-pressure receptors. When the venous pressure falls, the walls of the veins, atria and pulmonary vessels become less stretched. Sensory nerve endings detect this diminution in stretch, lessening sory nerve endings detect this diminution in stretch, lessening the the barrage of impulses to the sympathetic centre. This results in constriction of the resistance vessels and an increase in systemic vascular resistance, avoiding the fall in arterial pressure which would otherwise occur. This mechanism is important in changes of posture.

Higher centres of the brain. Other regions of the brain, including the cerebral cortex, affect the sympathetic centre. Thus excitement or anxiety stimulate the sympathetic centre, increasing the activity of the nerves to the heart and the peripheral circulation. Anyone who has sat an examination or run a race will remember the pounding of the heart which occurs even before the action begins.

In the peripheral circulation the effects of these control centres may be overridden by *local chemical effects* on blood vessels. The effects of changes in PO_2, PCO_2, lactic acid and adrenaline have already been described; many other chemical substances may be involved.

The effects of posture

If reflex adjustments did not occur, a change from the lying to the standing position would result in pooling of blood in the lower parts of the body, reduced venous return to the heart, lowered cardiac output and fainting. However, the diminished venous return of blood is detected by the low-pressure receptors and any change in arterial pressure by the baroreceptors; fewer impulses are sent from these receptors. Output from the vasomotor centre increases resulting in constriction of the resistance vessels, especially in those regions with a rich sympathetic innervation. As a result the blood flow to the lower part of the body is diminished, the systemic vascular resistance is increased and the arterial pressure is maintained. Because the arteries to the brain and heart muscle do not constrict, good flow is maintained to these organs. As already described, there is a simultaneous change in heart rate; you can check this by counting your pulse while lying down and again immediately after standing.

Sympathetic constriction of the arteries is associated with constriction of veins. Standing therefore constricts the veins in the legs, reducing the volume of the venous bed and increasing (or at least preventing a fall in) the venous return to the heart. Compression of veins by surrounding muscles (the 'muscle pump', p. 54) can also be important. Some people faint when standing for a long time on a hot day. They are less likely to do so if they regularly contract their leg muscles and so stimulate venous return. Pressure on abdominal veins by surrounding organs is increased on standing, and this also helps to maintain venous return to the heart.

EFFECTS OF ABNORMAL CONDITIONS ON THE HEART AND CIRCULATION

The heart

Abnormalities of conduction

We have already traced the conduction pathway through the normal heart (p. 41). Sometimes the passage of the excitation wave through the A–V node or bundle of His is blocked, and when none of the impulses get through to the ventricles this is called *complete heart block*. Damage to both right and left bundles has the same effect. Part of the conducting tissue distal to the block will then usually assume the role of pacemaker, at a rate lower than that of

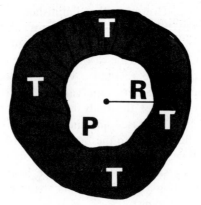

Fig. 9 Cross section of the left ventricle. By the law of Laplace tension in the ventricular wall (T) = pressure in the chamber (P) × half the radius of the chamber $\frac{R}{2}$.

the sinus node. Furthermore there is often very little increase in rate with sympathetic stimulation so that the cardiac output cannot increase as required during exercise, cardiac failure or haemorrhage.

Valve disease

There is practically no drop in pressure as blood flows through a normal valve but if the valve is narrowed a pressure gradient results. For instance, in severe *aortic stenosis*, systolic pressures might be LV 180, aorta 100; or in *pulmonary stenosis* RV 150, PA 20 mmHg. In each case a murmur is heard in systole as blood is pumped through the narrowed valve. Similarly in *mitral stenosis* there is a gradient across the mitral valve in diastole so that the mean diastolic pressure in the left atrium might be 15 mmHg, and in the left ventricle 5 mmHg. The heart chamber which must pump blood through the obstructed region is overworked and therefore hypertrophied.

If the mitral valve fails to close properly during systole (*mitral incompetence*) some blood will regurgitate from the left ventricle to the left atrium producing a systolic murmur. Pressure in the left atrium, and in the pulmonary veins entering it, rises. If the aortic valve does not close properly during diastole (*aortic incompetence*), some blood will leak back from the aorta to the left ventricle, producing a diastolic murmur. Since two thirds or more of the blood ejected with each beat may leak back in this way, the left ventricle must dilate to accommodate the extra volume and the myocardium must hypertrophy. It is an instructive exercise to work out which part of the heart is overloaded with other valvar defects.

The build up of pressure in the ventricle and ejection of blood result from contraction of muscle fibres and the development of *tension* in the wall of the ventricle. The relationship between this tension, the pressure generated and the size of the cardiac chamber are described by the Law of Laplace (Fig. 9).

$$\text{Tension} = \text{pressure} \times \frac{\text{radius}}{2}$$

Where a greater pressure is required (as in hypertension or aortic stenosis) greater tension must be generated. Similarly, if the ventricle becomes dilated (as in aortic incompetence), greater tension

must be generated to maintain the same pressure. High pressure
and dilatation of the ventricular chamber are the factors which
increase the oxygen demands of the myocardium and eventually
cause it to fail.

Intracardiac communications

Where an intracardiac communication is present a left to right shunt
occurs. Pressure in the left atrium is higher than that in the right
atrium because the left ventricle, with its thicker muscular wall, is
harder to fill. With an *atrial septal defect* (ASD) blood therefore
flows from the left to the right atrium. This blood, together with the
normal venous return, must be pumped through the lungs by the
right ventricle and pulmonary flow may be greatly increased. *Total
anomalous pulmonary venous return* amounts to a massive left to
right shunt at atrial level, all pulmonary venous blood returning by
one route or another to the right atrium.

Pressures in the left ventricle and aorta are higher than those in
the right ventricle and pulmonary artery because systemic vascular
resistance is higher than pulmonary vascular resistance (p. 50).
With a *ventricular septal defect* (VSD) or *patent ductus arteriosus*
(PDA), therefore, a left to right shunt also occurs. In these cases,
however, it is the left ventricle which bears the brunt of the extra
work load. In some more complex anomalies the functional disturbance is very similar to that seen in a VSD. In *double outlet right
ventricle* a VSD is present but both great arteries arise from the right
ventricle. If the VSD is large and close to the aortic valve, the
circulatory disturbance is really identical to that produced by a VSD
alone. In various forms of *single ventricle* there is effectively very
little ventricular septum at all but, provided the heart valves and
great arterial relationships are normal, the circulatory disturbance
is again very similar to that of a VSD. In practice valvar anomalies
(particularly mitral and pulmonary stenosis) are common and the
great arteries may be transposed.

Where pulmonary stenosis is associated with a VSD, as in *tetralogy of Fallot*, the situation is changed because blood in the right
ventricle may find an easier exit through the VSD to the aorta than
through the narrowed pulmonary valve. Venous blood then enters
the aorta and the patient is cyanosed. If the pulmonary valve is
totally *atretic*, venous blood can not enter the pulmonary artery

directly but must shunt right to left through a VSD or ASD. Except in the rare cases where there are large collateral vessels from the aorta passing directly to the lungs, blood reaches the lungs only through the PDA, and the patient can only survive as long as ductal flow, and therefore pulmonary blood flow, are sufficiently high to allow enough oxygen uptake from the lungs to support life.

Other patients are cyanosed because there is a direct anatomic connection between the right ventricle and the aorta. The most obvious example is *transposition of the great arteries* where the pulmonary and systemic circulations are independent; pulmonary venous blood passes to the left atrium and left ventricle in the normal way but then enters the pulmonary artery and returns to the lungs. Systemic venous drainage passes to the right atrium and right ventricle but then enters the aorta and returns around the body. Both pulmonary and systemic flows are often quite high but oxygen can only get to the systemic circuit through a patent ductus or an intracardiac communication. If no VSD is present the baby will rarely survive unassisted when the ductus begins to close, but balloon septostomy at cardiac catheterisation will usually allow adequate intracardiac mixing of the circulations to allow reasonable progress at least for a few months.

Cardiac failure

We have already seen that under normal circumstances the cardiac output can be varied to match the needs of the body. Circumstances may however arise in which the heart is unable to do this. Such failure may occur abruptly, for example when a large venous blood clot from a leg or the pelvis lodges in the main pulmonary artery. This is called *massive pulmonary embolism*. The right ventricle is unable to pump blood past the clot, the cardiac output immediately falls and death often follows rapidly. Less catastrophic but nevertheless rapid and severe failure may occur after an extensive myocardial infarction or after operation on a badly disordered heart. The effects of such acute cardiac failure are described in later sections.

Chronic cardiac failure develops when cardiac muscle which has been damaged (e.g. by repeated myocardial infarctions) is unable to cope with ordinary requirements. It also occurs when a basically healthy myocardium is no longer capable or working against such additional loads as are imposed by hypertension, valvar defects and intracardiac communications. In practice the heart tolerates extra *volume loads* quite well; with an ASD, for instance, the right ventricle may cope with a pulmonary flow which is three times normal for forty years before failure develops. With a VSD the left ventricle may pump twice the normal volume for most of a life-time before failure occurs. On the other hand the *pressure load* imposed on the right ventricle by severe pulmonary stenosis or pulmonary hypertension, or on the left ventricle by severe aortic stenosis or systemic hypertension, cannot be carried for so long.

In severe pulmonary stenosis or pulmonary hypertension *right ventricular failure* occurs. The right ventricle has difficulty in maintaining an adequate output and the pressure rises in the systemic veins. This increased filling pressure helps the right ventricle but it causes congestion in the abdominal organs with resultant anorexia, nausea and liver enlargement. Pressure in the capillaries rises, and sooner or later this pressure exceeds the osmotic pressure of the plasma proteins (p. 8). At this point fluid begins to escape from the capillaries into the interstitial tissues and oedema develops, particularly in the most dependant parts of the body. Oedema develops more readily in patients with low levels of protein in the plasma.

In ischaemic heart disease, systemic hypertension or disease of the aortic valve *left ventricular failure* occurs. Pulmonary venous pressure rises, the lungs become congested and the patient becomes breathless. In severe cases pulmonary oedema develops; fluid escapes from the capillaries into interstitial tissues and alveoli. The patient with pulmonary oedema becomes extremely breathless, has to sit up in his struggle for air and may cough copious, frothy sputum which is sometimes tinged with blood. In the chest x-ray fluffy shadows due to oedema can be seen in the lungs. The presence of fluid in the alveoli prevents adequate oxygenation of the blood and the patient may die of asphyxia.

With either left- or right-sided failure secondary effects, largely due to reduced cardiac output, occur. There is a general rise in systemic vascular resistance, particularly in organs such as the kidneys. Reduced renal perfusion leads to increased production of renin with a consequent increased release of angiotensin and aldosterone:

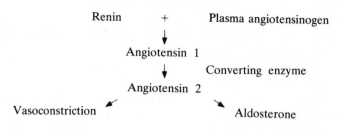

Vasoconstriction is therefore accentuated and the increased production of aldosterone leads to retention by the kidneys of sodium and water with the result that fluid gradually accumulates in the extra cellular space. This aggravates congestion of the lungs and systemic tissues. Failure of either side of the heart thus leads progressively to a condition of persistently low output, somewhat raised systemic vascular resistance, with pulmonary and systemic congestion, and this is the state of *congestive heart failure.* Treatment must be directed to increasing the efficiency of the heart with digoxin and other inotropic drugs, and increasing the urinary excretion of sodium and water with diuretics. The work of the overloaded ventricle may be reduced by the administration of vasodilating drugs. Emergency measures may be required to relieve pulmonary oedema.

The peripheral circulation: the effects of haemorrhage

If about 1 litre of blood is lost by haemorrhage, the veins and arteries are less well filled and the pressure will start to fall in both. Poor filling of the veins leads to a fall in cardiac output and if this effect were added to the fall in arterial pressure due to underfilling it would not be possible to maintain perfusion to vital areas such as the heart and brain. However, the mechanisms already described act to minimize these harmful changes, as follows.

Primary change. Fall in arterial pressure, venous pressure and cardiac output.

Immediate result. Decrease in impulses from high-pressure and low-pressure receptors to:
1 The parasympathetic centre.
2 The sympathetic centre.

Motor response.
1   Reduction in vagal activity, with an increase in heart rate.
2   Increase in sympathetic activity.
a   Increase in heart rate.
b   More efficient ventricular contraction.
c   Constriction of resistance vessels, especially in the skin, kidneys and spleen.
d   Generalized constriction of capacitance vessels, with improved filling of the heart.
e   Stimulation of the adrenal glands to release adrenaline and noradrenaline into the circulation.

These changes minimize the fall in arterial pressure and cardiac output. There is, of course, a limit to the compensation which can be achieved and death will result if loss of blood is massive. Nor can the patient survive indefinitely in a critical, barely compensated state because secondary effects develop, described later in the section on shock (p. 192).

The pulmonary circulation: effects of cardiac abnormalities

Cardiac abnormalities have important effects on the lung which must be mentioned briefly.
1   With a large left-to-right shunt, pulmonary flow and the volume of blood in the lungs are both very high. Radiologically the pulmonary arteries look overfilled with blood, an appearance described as *plethora*. With left ventricular failure or a high left atrial pressure due to mitral valve disease, pressure is high in the pulmonary veins and capillaries and the lungs become *congested*. With both plethora and congestion the lungs are stiff, turgid with blood and susceptible to infection. With bronchitis or pneumonia the problems of infection are added to these changes and the patient may rapidly become very ill.
2   With a large ventricular septal defect or patent ductus blood is pumped through the lungs not only at a high flow rate but also at a high pressure. Some patients respond with a marked increase in pulmonary vascular resistance. This cuts down the flow through the lungs and may bring about an improvement in the patient's condition. Such a reaction is not, however, without disadvantage, since the risks of surgical correction increase when the pulmonary vascu-

lar resistance is high. Indeed if the resistance is too high the condition may be inoperable.

A similar reaction is shown by some patients with mitral valve disease. Pulmonary venous congestion is then minimized but it becomes very difficult for the right ventricle to pump blood through the lungs. The patient cannot increase his output with exercise and his activity is consequently very limited. Sooner or later he may go into congestive cardiac failure. Fortunately this response is reversible if the valve disease can be cured surgically but the limited cardiac output and congestive failure may considerably increase the risks of the immediate postoperative period.

The pulmonary resistance-vessels in infants are much more muscular than those of older patients and an increased pulmonary vascular resistance is seen much more commonly in the first year of life. Mitral valve disease is of course uncommon at this age, and high resistance problems are usually associated with left-to-right shunts. Although the resistance will usually fall gradually after surgical correction, the immediate postoperative period may again be very difficult. The muscular resistance-vessels constrict vigorously in response to hypoxia, acidosis and high P_{CO_2} levels. In the management of young infants, therefore, it is particularly important to maintain good ventilation and satisfactory P_{O_2} levels, and to avoid acidosis.

4 Respiration

Life demands the production and expenditure of energy, even under resting conditions. The cells generate energy by 'burning' (i.e. oxidizing) carbohydrate or fat (p. 19), and in the process consume oxygen (O_2) and produce carbon dioxide (CO_2). The rate at which the cells carry on this exchange of O_2 for CO_2 depends upon the energy requirement. It is increased, for example, by exercise, fever, hyperthyroidism and trauma, including surgical trauma. It is reduced by hypothermia and hypothyroidism. The lungs are the means by which O_2 is supplied, and CO_2 eliminated, at a rate appropriate to the body's needs.

Anatomy (Fig. 10)

The lungs consist of a conducting airway and a region of gas-exchange. They may be described as follows:

1 *The upper airway:* mouth, nose, pharynx.

2 *The lower airway:* larynx, trachea, left and right main bronchi, lobar bronchi and segmental bronchi down to terminal bronchioles. The branched structure of the airway gives rise to the term 'bronchial tree', whose finest 'twigs' are only 0.2 mm in diameter.

3 *The alveoli (singular, 'alveolus'):* These are the tiny air-spaces which make up most of the lung volume. Their thin walls contain a dense network of capillary blood-vessels through which blood passes from the pulmonary artery to the pulmonary veins. The blood in the capillaries is almost in contact with the alveolar gas, and exchange of O_2 and CO_2 between gas and blood can normally occur very easily.

The large airways have rings of cartilage in their walls which help to keep them open. Narrower bronchi contain less cartilage and bronchioles none; but as cartilage diminishes there is an increase in muscle, disposed in rings and spirals in the wall of the airway. This

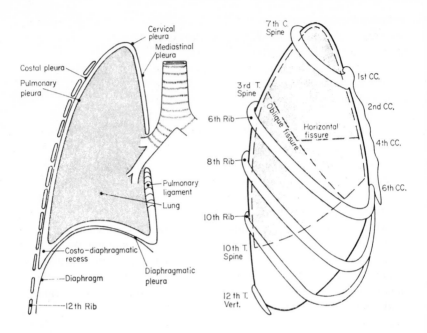

Fig. 10 Anatomy of the lungs. Left, section viewed from front. Right, lateral view of the right lung, pleura and ribs. From *A Companion to Medical Studies*, vol. I (1968).

muscle can contract, narrowing the small airways, and is under the control of the autonomic nervous system (p. 32). Bronchiolar muscle also contracts in response to histamine and other substances, and allergic reactions may thus include bronchoconstriction.

The trachea and bronchi are lined with a layer of cells which have a brushlike surface consisting of fine filaments called *cilia*; the cilia are in constant motion, sweeping mucus, dust and bacteria up the airway towards the pharynx. They are an important part of the defences against inhaled particles, but are readily put out of action by irritant vapours, drying or inflammation.

Each lung is invested with two layers of a thin membrane, the *pleura*, rather as a fist, pushed into the side of a closed and empty plastic bag would be invested by the plastic. The 'space' between the layers is lubricated by a thin film of serous liquid. The inner layer is firmly adherent to the lung, the outer layer to the inside of the thoracic wall and the sides of the mediastinum. During inflation and deflation of the lungs the pleural layers slide easily on one another. The main bronchi and the pulmonary arteries and veins occupy the 'necks' of the two pleural 'bags'.

The thoracic cavity containing the lungs and pleura is bounded in front, behind and laterally by the ribs and intercostal muscles, below by the diaphragm and medially by the heart and other mediastinal structures.

The mechanics of breathing

Breathing requires work (we speak of 'laboured breathing'!) and work implies a force ('resistance') against which work is done. The forces which must be overcome in breathing are of two kinds. One of these arises from the fact that both the lungs and the thoracic cage are *elastic* structures; that is, they tend to resist deformation and, when inflated or deflated from a position of equilibrium, they return to this position when the displacing force has been removed. The other kind of force is *frictional*, and is set up whenever air is moved through the airway.

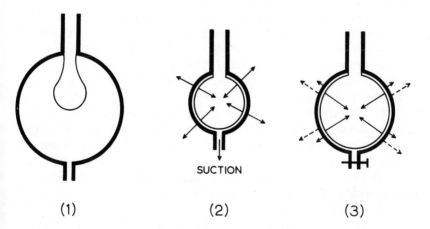

Fig. 11 The forces acting on the lungs and thorax. For description, see text.

Elastic forces and 'elastic work'. When a needle is pushed into the pleural 'space', air enters to form a pneumothorax; at the same time the lungs contract and the thorax expands. If the air is sucked out again the lungs expand and the thorax contracts.

Fig. 11 shows the forces acting on the lungs and thorax. At (1), the relaxed or equilibrium positions of the lungs and thorax separately are shown, with a space between them full of air at atmospheric pressure. In this position there are no elastic forces. If now the air is pumped out of the space between the lungs and thorax (2) the lungs expand and the thorax becomes smaller; elastic forces develop, as though the lungs were trying to shrink and the thorax trying to expand. These forces are shown as arrows, and in the new, combined equilibrium position they balance each other. The pleural 'space' lies between these opposing forces and the pressure within it must therefore be 'negative' i.e. less than atmospheric. In (3), an extra force has been added, shown by the dashed arrows; this is the force exerted by the muscles of inspiration. It upsets the balance shown in (2), and causes the lungs and thorax to expand. As the lungs expand, their elastic force of recoil increases, and in (3) their arrows are longer to illustrate this. On the other hand the thorax, being nearer to its own equilibrium position (1) is less 'strained', and its elastic arrows are therefore shorter in (3). The elastic forces are thus unequal, but the difference has been made up by the muscular force. Note that the total forces pulling against each other are now greater than in (2), and the 'intrapleural' pressure is therefore more 'negative' in position (3). Removal of the muscular force would again imbalance the forces, and the lungs would pull the thorax inwards until position (2) was regained.

We may summarize the above, in terms of the real lungs and thorax, as follows:

1 The lungs and thorax, being elastic structures, normally exert a pull on each other. In the absence of other forces (e.g. muscular) a position is reached in which the opposing forces are balanced.

2 Because of these opposing forces, the pressure within the pleural 'space' is 'negative', i.e. subatmospheric. This is the pressure to which all the thoracic contents are exposed, and it is termed the *intrathoracic pressure.*

3 To inflate the lungs an extra force must be applied by the muscles of inspiration.

4 During inflation, intrathoracic pressure falls still further.

5 Expiration is normally almost wholly 'passive', i.e. it is achieved by the elastic forces returning to a balanced position.
6 Expiration can be active, as in forced breathing. In this case the expiratory muscles assist the elastic forces to bring about a more rapid deflation.

The inspiratory muscles, in upsetting the balance of elastic forces, do mechanical work; the greater the depth of breathing, the more of this 'elastic work' must be done.

The ease with which the chest and lungs can be expanded is called the *compliance*. It is measured as the change in the volume of the lungs in response to a change in pressure. Normal chest and lung compliance is about 1 litre per kPa (100 ml per cmH$_2$O). This figure is smaller if the lungs are stiff and larger when the lungs are very elastic.

Frictional forces and 'frictional work'. The heat generated between wood and sandpaper is due to work done against the force of friction; this force appears as soon as the sandpaper begins to move. In the same way, the flow of air through a tube sets up frictional forces, and a small but measurable amount of work must be done to maintain the flow. Frictional forces and frictional work in breathing are therefore not necessarily dependent on the depth of breathing but rather on the speed with which air moves through the airway.

Factors which increase the work of breathing

Congestion of the pulmonary vessels, consolidation of the lung (as in pneumonia), and pulmonary infiltration with fibrous or other tissue all decrease lung compliance—that is to say a bigger muscular force is needed to produce a given degree of inflation. Loss of pulmonary tissue has the same effect, for the remaining lung must be stretched more to accommodate the same tidal volume. All these conditions increase 'elastic work'. Frictional work is increased when the airways are narrowed and this is very obvious in an attack of asthma. Rapid, shallow breathing also needs more frictional work than slow, deep breathing.

Surface tension of the alveoli

The surface tension of isotonic saline is high and if isotonic saline lined the alveoli a pressure of 70 cm H_2O would be required just to keep them open. When the surface tension is constant a small bubble needs a higher pressure to keep it open than does a large one. If this happened in the lungs all small alveoli would collapse. Pulmonary *surfactant* is a lipoprotein which lines the alveoli and produces a marked reduction in the surface tension. It also has the property of decreasing the surface tension even further as an alveolus gets smaller. Deficiency or absence of surfactant leads to atelectasis and decreased compliance. Surfactant is deficient in the lungs of premature infants. Pulmonary oedema and prolonged administration of high oxygen concentrations lead to surfactant deficiency. Surfactant is also depleted in many other lung diseases.

The respiratory muscles

Inspiratory muscles. The *intercostal muscles* raise the ribs to a more horizontal position, and swing them outwards like bucket handles. In this way the size of the thorax is increased from back to front and also from side to side. The *diaphragm,* when it contracts, enlarges the chest vertically and also, in health, raises and widens the lower ribs; if the diaphragm is not domed but flat, as in emphysema, it draws the lower ribs inwards.

Expiratory muscles. The main expiratory muscles are those of the abdominal wall. Expiration is of course, normally passive at rest.

The accessory muscles of respiration. These are muscles of the neck, shoulders and trunk which, when called upon, can contribute to respiratory movements by raising the ribs or compressing the abdomen. The most important are the muscles of the abdominal wall which can push the relaxed diaphragm upwards, thus causing a powerful expiratory movement.

Paralysis of the respiratory muscles may be due to disease (e.g. polyneuritis) or to muscle-relaxing drugs such as tubocurarine.

The intrathoracic pressure

During ordinary breathing the intrathoracic pressure is 'negative', varying in different parts of the pleural space from $-0\cdot3$ to $-1\cdot3$ kPa ($-2\cdot5$ to -10 mmHg). In any one person the pressure drop from expiration to inspiration is about 0·3 kPa (2·5 mmHg). The thin central veins and atria are exposed to the intrathoracic pressure and its 'negativity' favours the return of blood to the right heart. The intrathoracic pressure may, however, be raised to above atmospheric by the following:

1 *An expiratory effort against a closed glottis* (Valsalva manoeuvre) causes an inward force on the chest wall which exceeds the elastic force of recoil of the lungs, and the intrathoracic pressure swings to the 'positive' side so long as the effort continues. This can be made use of when pleural drainage tubes have to be removed, to prevent air entering the pleural space through the hole left by the tube; the patient maintains the Valsalva effort until the stitch has been tied to seal the hole. *Violent coughing* may increase intrathoracic pressure by as much as 13 kPa (100 mmHg).

2 *Intermittent positive pressure ventilation* (IPPV) reverses the normal pressure-cycle in the chest (p. 255). At the end of expiration the mean intrathoracic pressure is still (say) $-0·7$ kPa (-5 mmHg), but when the lungs are inflated it rises to about $+0·7$ kPa ($+5$ mmHg). The chief consequence is that venous return to the right heart is impeded and venous pressure increases by up to 0·7 kPa (5 mmHg). This does not imply cardiac failure. Because the increased intrathoracic pressure compresses the heart, the cardiac muscle fibres are less stretched and the cardiac stroke volume is decreased (p. 48). This also occurs when the pressure around the heart is increased by *cardiac tamponade* (p. 189). The decreased stretch of the atrial muscle fibres is detected by the low pressure receptors resulting in an increased systemic vascular resistance (p. 56) and the secretion of aldosterone (p. 12). The aldosterone effect is one of the mechanisms leading to fluid retention during intermittent positive pressure ventilation.

Summary

The mechanical properties of the airway, lungs and thorax are important in two respects: (1) Mechanical work is done in stretching the lungs and in pushing air along the bronchi and bronchioles, and it is increased in various abnormalities of the lungs. (2) The mechanics of the lungs and thorax result in a subatmospheric (or 'negative') intrathoracic pressure, which is an important factor assisting venous return to the heart.

Pulmonary ventilation

Fig. 12 illustrates the principle of gas exchange between lungs and atmosphere and the mechanism of pulmonary ventilation. At stage (1) inspiration is about to begin; the lungs (including the airway) are full of gas which has given up some of its oxygen (O_2) and take up carbon dioxide (CO_2). Waiting to enter the airway is a volume of inspired air, which is shown as three times the volume of the airway. On inspiration (2) this air drives the spent gas, which occupies the airway, back into the alveoli and a quantity of fresh air also reaches the alveoli. At the end of inspiration the airway is full of inspired fresh air (one 'unit') and thus two 'units' must have entered the alveoli. Next (3) these two units lose some O_2 and take up CO_2, becoming like the rest of the gas in the alveoli (which is termed *alveolar gas*). Lastly (4) expiration occurs; alveolar gas drives out the 'unit' of inspired air (which is unchanged) and two units of alveolar gas also escape from the airway, leaving the airway full of alveolar gas. This is the situation in stage (1), and another cycle begins. Three 'units' of air have been inspired, and three 'units' of expired gas have been expired; the latter consist of two 'units' of

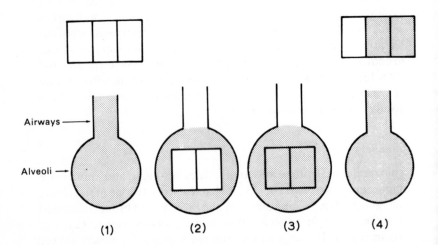

Fig. 12   Alveolar gas exchange. See text.

alveolar gas mixed with one 'unit' of fresh air which had remained unchanged in the airway. The whole process is, of course, continuous, but is easier to describe in stages.

In the above account the 'unit' of volume chosen was the volume of the conducting airway, about 150 ml, and the tidal volume was taken for convenience as 450 ml. These are roughly normal for an adult at rest. Since the air which passed no further than the airways did not exchange O_2 for CO_2 with the blood, this part of the respiratory tract is called the *deadspace*. Of every breath taken, between $\frac{1}{4}$ and $\frac{1}{3}$ merely enters and leaves the deadspace. It follows that of the total gas entering the lungs each minute (the *ventilation rate* or *minute volume,* measured in l per min) only $\frac{2}{3}$ to $\frac{3}{4}$ is used for the purpose of gas exchange. If the total ventilation rate is 6 l per min, perhaps 4 l per min (the *alveolar ventilation* (*rate*)) is 'useful'. The remaining 2 l per min is the *deadspace ventilation* (*rate*) and in this respect is 'wasted'. The deadspace is however of considerable value in other ways. It humidifies and warms the air passing through it very efficiently; by the time the inspired air reaches the alveoli it is at body temperature and saturated with water vapour.

Control of ventilation rate

Alveolar ventilation is normally adjusted closely to the needs of the body for gas exchange. During exercise, for example, more O_2 is used, more CO_2 is produced, and alveolar ventilation increases proportionally. The regulation is made possible by receptors which are extremely sensitive to changes in the partial pressures of O_2 and CO_2 (p. 80). O_2 lack in the arterial blood stimulates receptors in the carotid bodies (tiny collections of cells near the carotid sinuses (p. 56) and a reflex is set up which increases ventilation. Excess of CO_2 stimulates receptors on the surface of the hind-brain inside the skull, and changes in CO_2 pressure in cerebrospinal fluid have an even greater effect than those in the blood. Increase in acidity also stimulates ventilation via the same receptors, and this is an important mechanism in compensating for acid-base upsets (p. 16). Ordinarily these three stimuli (O_2 lack, CO_2 excess and acidity) act together to regulate the ventilation; just as a ship's automatic pilot keeps it on course, so the breathing is normally regulated to keep the O_2 and CO_2 pressures, and the acid-base state, of the body fluids within narrow limits.

Control of respiratory frequency

The volume of each breath (*tidal volume*) multiplied by the number of breaths per min (*respiratory frequency*) equals the ventilation rate. It is clear that a given ventilation rate may be achieved by various combinations of tidal volume and frequency. How does the body decide which combination to use? Slow, deep breathing increases 'elastic' work and rapid, shallow breathing increases 'frictional' work (p. 70). There is an optimal frequency and volume at which total respiratory work is least, and the body seems to make just this compromise. How it does so is uncertain. Adjustments are often seen in disease. In pulmonary congestion, or any other state in which the lungs are abnormally stiff, tidal volume is sacrificed at the expense of frequency and respiration is rapid and shallow. When frictional work is increased, e.g. in asthma, breathing tends to be slow.

Distribution of inspired air

We have seen that about $\frac{1}{3}$ of the inspired air gets no further than the conducting airway. The remaining $\frac{2}{3}$ of each breath is normally distributed fairly evenly to the alveoli in different regions of the lung. In disease of the lung this is often not so, and some alveoli get less, others more, than their fair share of inspired air. This happens also, to some degree, when IPPV is substituted for natural breathing. For example, unless blood flow to overventilated alveoli is increased, some of the air reaching these alveoli cannot exchange with the blood and is 'wasted' just like the deadspace ventilation (Fig. 13). It follows that when a *ventilation-perfusion mismatch* of this nature occurs, the *effective* alveolar ventilation is less than the actual ventilation. This is why patients being mechanically ventilated need a 20–40 per cent greater ventilation than when breathing spontaneously. If this extra ventilation is not supplied, arterial $P\text{CO}_2$ will rise and $P\text{O}_2$ fall (p. 85).

Summary

Only part of the total pulmonary ventilation reaches the alveoli, where gas exchange takes place with the blood. About $\frac{1}{4}$ to $\frac{1}{3}$ of the ventilation simply enters and leaves the respiratory deadspace. The

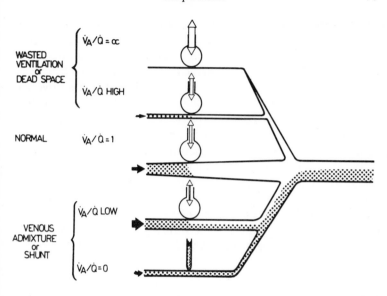

Fig. 13 Types of ventilation—perfusion abnormalities. The diagram illustrates how mismatching of ventilation (open arrows) and perfusion (dark arrows) leads to inefficient gas exchange. The best exchange occurs in areas of the lung where ventilation and perfusion are matched (centre of diagram). The upper part of the diagram represents well-ventilated but poorly or non-perfused areas of lung which lead to wasted ventilation, and the lower part represents well perfused but poorly or unventilated areas that cause venous admixture.

remaining $\frac{2}{3}$ to $\frac{3}{4}$ is normally used efficiently for gas exchange, but if unevenly distributed to alveoli part of it is 'wasted', as though it were deadspace ventilation.

Pulmonary blood-flow

This is the flow from pulmonary arteries to pulmonary veins, and normally amounts to about 5 l per min (the cardiac output, p. 48) at rest. As with ventilation, unevenness of blood flow occurs in many pulmonary diseases. If this results in mismatching of ventilation and perfusion, gas exchange becomes less efficient.

Blood leaving alveoli which are well perfused but poorly ventilated has a high PCO_2 and low PO_2. This type of mismatch is called *venous admixture* or *shunt* because its effect is the same as if some of the blood has been shunted from the right to the left side of the heart without passing through the lungs (Fig. 13). The opposite is the case with well-ventilated but poorly perfused alveoli. Accurately matched distribution changes (caused, for instance by pneumonectomy or pleural effusion, which affect ventilation and blood flow equally) result in only minor upsets in gas exchange.

The nature and magnitude of ventilation perfusion mismatches is described by the *ratio* of ventilation to perfusion ($\dot{V}_A/\dot{Q}$). A *high* ratio may be caused by an *increase* in ventilation or a *decrease* in perfusion to an area of lung and results in 'wasted' ventilation. Conversely a *low* ratio results from *decreased* ventilation or *increased* perfusion and the shunted blood leads to a lower than expected arterial PO_2.

Closing capacity

As a patient over about 60 years of age breathes out, a lung volume is reached at which the small airways in the lowermost areas of the lungs begin to close successively. The volume at which this process starts is called the *closing capacity* and it changes with posture and age. Teenagers and young adults have an end-expiratory lung volume greater than the closing capacity and do not have airway closure during normal breathing. It can, however, occur during forced expiration. As age increases the closing capacity increases until airway closure occurs during each tidal expiration and the affected lung regions suffer a reduction in ventilation. The same phenomenon occurs between birth and about 5 years of age. This is why arterial PO_2 is lower in infants and the elderly than in young adults. Pulmonary disease may decrease lung volume to less than closing capacity so that some airways are permanently closed during normal breathing; they open only with deep breathing or if the lung volume at end-expiration is increased. This increased volume can be achieved by means of positive end-expiratory pressure (PEEP) during intermittent positive pressure ventilation or by continuous positive airway pressure (CPAP, p. 257) during spontaneous breathing.

The carriage of gases in the blood

Before this can be understood it is necessary to know something about the *partial pressures of gases in solution.*

Atmospheric pressure

Fig. 14 shows a mercury-in-glass barometer. The height of the column of mercury in the barometer is AB. Above A, there is a vacuum. The pressure at B is therefore entirely due to the weight of the column AB. Since B and C lie at the same horizontal level and are connected by a stationary liquid (mercury), the pressure at C equals the pressure at B. The pressure at C is due to the weight of the atmosphere, and the height AB is therefore a measure of atmospheric pressure. This is why atmospheric pressure, or any pressure, can be expressed in millimetres of mercury (mmHg). In many countries it still is; however the unit of pressure agreed in Europe (SI, Appendix 6) is the kiloPascal (kPa). 1 mmHg equals

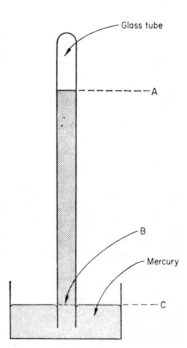

Fig. 14 Diagram of a barometer. Mercury extends up the glass tube to A. Above this is a vacuum. Pressure at B is equal to pressure at C, since they are on the same level. See text.

0·133 kPa. (Circulatory pressures are still given in mmHg.) At sea level, standard atmospheric (or 'barometric') pressure is 101 kPa (760 mmHg) but the actual pressure varies with humidity and other meteorological conditions.

Partial pressure of gas

Atmospheric air consists of 20·94 per cent O_2, 0·03 per cent CO_2 and 79·03 per cent nitrogen (N_2) by volume. If the barometric pressure is 101 kPa (760 mmHg) we can visualize this as being made up of *partial pressures* due to the constituent gases. The partial pressure of O_2 (PO_2) would be 20·94 per cent of 101, or about 21 kPa (159 mmHg), the PN_2 79·03 per cent of 101, or about 80 kPa (600 mmHg) and the PCO_2 0·03 kPa (0·2 mmHg). All the partial pressures add up to 101 kP (760 mmHg). When air is inspired, water vapour is added to it from the walls of the deadspace and since water vapour is a gas, it has its own partial pressure (6·3 kPa (47 mmHg) at full humidity and 37°C). Four gases thus enter the alveoli:

		Partial pressure	
Gas		(mmHg)	(kPa)
Water vapour		47·0	6·3
Oxygen	(20·94 per cent of 760 − 47)	149·3	19·9
Nitrogen	(79·03 per cent of 760 − 47)	563·5	75·1
Carbon dioxide	(0·03 per cent of 760 − 47)	0·2	0·03
Totals	100·00 per cent	760·0	101·3

Breathing air, the inspired PO_2 is thus about 20 kPa (150 mmHg) and the inspired PCO_2 practically zero. Breathing 100 per cent O_2, the alveoli receive only O_2 and water vapour, and PO_2 is thus 100 per cent of $(101 − 6·3)$, or 94·7 kPa (713 mmHg). For these calculations a barometric pressure of 101 kPa (760 mmHg) has been assumed.

Gases in solution

Most gases dissolve in water. The amount of gas which dissolves in a given volume of water depends on the *solubility* of the gas and upon the *partial pressure* of the gas to which the liquid is exposed.

1 The solubility depends upon the particular gas; CO_2 is much more soluble than O_2. Solubility also varies with temperature, and all gases become less soluble as temperature rises; we make water air-free by boiling it.

2 The greater the partial pressure of a gas, the more of it can be held in solution in a given liquid. Use is made of this fact in the manufacture of soda-water, which is a solution of CO_2 in water at a partial pressure of 2 or 3 atmospheres. When a bottle of soda-water is opened and thus exposed to a pressure of only 1 atmosphere, most of the dissolved CO_2 comes out of solution and appears in the liquid as bubbles. We can thus visualize, in an unopened soda-water bottle, a partial pressure of CO_2 in both the liquid and the gas above the liquid; at equilibrium these two pressures are equal. When a mixture of gases goes into solution, each constituent gas (e.g. O_2, N_2 or CO_2) behaves as if it alone were present at its particular partial pressure. Gases enter and leave the blood strictly in accordance with differences in their partial pressures between the blood and the outside of the capillary vessel.

It is important to distinguish between the *partial pressure* of a gas and the *concentration* of a gas in solution. If O_2 and CO_2 are dissolved in water at the same partial pressure, about 20 times as much CO_2 as O_2 will be present. This is because CO_2 is much more soluble than O_2. By contrast, in a *gas mixture* containing O_2 and CO_2 at the same partial pressure, the concentrations of O_2 and CO_2 are also equal.

Units of measurement. Partial pressure is measured in kPa (see also Appendix 6) and denoted by the symbol *P*—thus PO_2, PCO_2. Concentration of a gas is measured as ml of gas per 100 ml of liquid. Since the number of ml of gas would depend on the temperature and pressure at which its volume is measured, we use the volume the gas would have at 101 kPa (760 mmHg) and 0°C, dry.

The blood gases

Since blood comes regularly in contact with alveolar gas, it contains O_2, N_2 and CO_2 which are all soluble. In addition it holds O_2 and CO_2 (but not N_2) in easily reversible chemical combination, and thus contains much more O_2 and CO_2 than could be accounted for on the basis of solubility alone. We have seen that for either O_2 or CO_2 there is a simple relationship between partial pressure and concentration of dissolved gas. The concentration of chemically combined O_2 and CO_2 is also related to PCO_2 and PO_2, but the relationship is not a simple one.

Oxygen

Combined O_2. Red cells contain a pigment, haemoglobin, which has the unique property of combining loosely with O_2. The chemical reaction can be written:

Hb	+	$4O_2$	$\rightleftharpoons$	Hb $(O_2)_4$
(reduced) haemoglobin		oxygen		oxyhaemoglobin
blue-purple				red

The arrows in this equation point both ways, showing that the reaction is reversible; oxyhaemoglobin can release O_2, becoming reduced haemoglobin in the process.

One molecule of haemoglobin can combine with one, two, three or four molecules of O_2, and there are millions of haemoglobin molecules in each red cell. It is therefore possible for blood to hold, at any given moment, less than its full quota of O_2 in combination; the 'full quota' must obviously depend on the amount of haemoglobin present. Normally, blood contains 15 g of haemoglobin per 100 ml. This amount of haemoglobin can combine with 20 ml of O_2 when 'fully (or 100 per cent) saturated', and this is called the O_2 *capacity* of that particular sample of blood. A patient with only 7·5 g of haemoglobin per 100 ml has an O_2 capacity of half this, namely 10 ml O_2 per 100 ml. On the other hand, a blood sample may have an O_2 *content* which is less than the O_2 capacity; it may be 25, 50, 80 or any other percentage of the capacity, and is then spoken of as 'undersaturated' or 'unsaturated' with O_2. 'Desaturated' usually implies that there is no combined O_2 at all. All these terms are, however, rather loosely used.

The colour of blood depends upon its degree of saturation with O_2. It becomes noticeably blue at about 85 per cent and at 70 per cent is decidedly blue. One method of measuring saturation accurately uses a photocell to detect 'redness' in the blood sample. When arterial blood is less than 85 per cent saturated with oxygen, its blueness commonly gives rise to the clinical sign of *cyanosis*. In this case the cyanosis is described as *central,* because the arterial blood is already abnormal before it reaches the tissues. When peripheral blood-flow is reduced, the skin, especially of the hands, ears and nose, may become blue even if arterial blood is normal; the blueness reflects the extra depletion of oxygen in the venous blood in the skin. The part is cooler than normal, because its blood flow is diminished. This type of cyanosis is termed *peripheral,* and is common in states of low cardiac output. Both central and peripheral factors may be involved in a given patient with cyanosis.

The way in which PO_2 affects percentage saturation is shown by the *oxyhaemoglobin dissociation curve* (Fig. 15). This is S-shaped, and has a steep part between PO_2 3 and PO_2 8 kPa (20 and 60 mmHg. Further increase in PO_2 causes less and less increase in saturation, and from 13 kPa (100 mmHg) upwards the saturation can increase by only about 5 per cent, from 95 to 100. Arterial blood

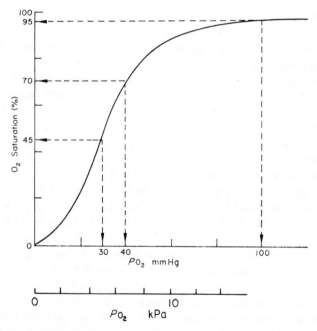

Fig. 15 The 'dissociation curve' of oxyhaemoglobin. Normal arterial blood is 95 to 98 per cent saturated, and normal mixed venous blood about 70 per cent saturated with oxygen.

normally has a PO_2 of about 13 kPa (100 mmHg), saturation 95 per cent, content 95 per cent of 20 ml per 100 ml or 19 ml of O_2 per 100 ml of blood (assuming a haemoglobin concentration of 15 g per 100 ml). Mixed venous PO_2 is about 5·3 kPa (40 mmHg), saturation 70 per cent, content 70 per cent of 20 ml per 100 ml or 14 ml O_2 per 100 ml. The *arteriovenous O_2 difference* is thus 19 minus 14, or 5 ml O_2 per 100 ml blood; this is the volume of O_2 given up to the tissues by every 100 ml of blood.

It will be obvious that since the venous blood still has 70 per cent of its O_2 capacity unused, there is a large reserve available for emergencies. As an example we may consider what happens when *cardiac output* falls. A normal output of 5 l per min can be thought of as 50 units of 100 ml each. These provide the tissues with 50 times 5 ml of O_2, or 250 ml per min which is the normal O_2 uptake. If output is halved, only 25 units of 100 ml of blood are available to the tissues each minute. To maintain O_2 uptake, each unit must give up twice as much O_2, or 10 ml O_2, to the tissues ($25 \times 10 = 250$). The arteriovenous O_2 difference thus increases from 5 to 10 ml per 100 ml. The venous blood then contains 19 minus 10, or 9 ml of O_2 per 100 ml, and its O_2 saturation is $\frac{9}{20}$, or 45 per cent. There is still some reserve, but it has been reduced. From the dissociation curve we see that at 45 per cent the PO_2 is about 4 kPa (30 mmHg), only 1·3 kPa (10 mmHg) less than it was. A little arithmetic will show that cardiac output would have to fall to about 1·3 l/min before all the O_2 in arterial blood need be extracted by the tissues.

In these calculations we have assumed that haemoglobin concentration is normal. *Anaemia* must now be considered. Suppose haemoglobin concentration is halved from 15 to 7·5 g per 100 ml. This halves the O_2 capacity from 20 to 10 ml per 100 ml, and an arterial saturation of 95 per cent would give a content of 9·5 instead of 19 ml per 100 ml. The loss of 5 ml per 100 ml in the tissues would then bring venous O_2 content to 4·5 ml per 100 ml, corresponding to a saturation of 4·5/10 or 45 per cent. This is the same result as we obtained by halving cardiac output, and indeed a reduction in either output or haemoglobin concentration act in the same way to reduce the total O_2 delivered to the tissues each minute. If the tissues continue to use the same amount of O_2 per minute, the reserve of O_2 in venous blood will be partly (or completely) used up. A combination of reduced output and anaemia is serious, for each multiplies the effects of the other.

Dissolved O_2. Blood dissolves only 0·0225 ml of O_2 per 100 ml of blood for every kPa of P_{O_2}. Thus normal arterial blood at a P_{O_2} of 13·3 kPa has 0·0225 × 13·3, or 0·3 ml of O_2 dissolved in every 100 ml of blood. This is a very small amount compared with the 19 ml of O_2 held in combination. Dissolved O_2 may however become important when P_{O_2} is increased, as when pure O_2 is increased, as when pure O_2 is breathed at atmospheric pressure (P_{O_2} about 80 kPa or 600 mmHg) or in a compression chamber at 3 atmospheres (P_{O_2} about 265 kPa or 2000 mmHg). In the latter case, dissolved O_2 concentration will be 0·0225 × 265, or 6 ml per 100 ml. This figure is actually bigger than the normal arteriovenous oxygen difference. Under these conditions combined O_2 is not used at all, and venous O_2 saturation (i.e. *combined* O_2) is the same as arterial. *High pressure ('hyperbaric') O_2* may thus be of use in treating arterial disease or vascular injuries because it helps to sustain the supply of O_2 to the tissues. Even when breathed at atmospheric pressure (dissolved O_2 0·0225 × 80 or 1·8 ml per 100 ml) pure oxygen increases dissolved O_2 to a useful level. It is thus worth administering in severe anaemia or shock (p. 192) since it helps to supplement the diminished amount of combined O_2 reaching the tissues per minute.

Carbon dioxide

Like O_2, CO_2 is present in blood in dissolved and combined forms. It is not however necessary to deal with these except to refer to the connection between P_{CO_2} and ventilatory failure (p. 87) and acidosis (p. 15). Normally arterial P_{CO_2} is about 5·3 kPa (40 mmHg) and mixed venous P_{CO_2} about 6·4 kPa (48 mmHg). The level of P_{CO_2} affects both dissolved and combined CO_2 content. As P_{CO_2} increases, CO_2 content continues to rise, and there is no levelling off in combined CO_2 as in the case of O_2.

The effect of pulmonary ventilation on the blood gases

Let us imagine a room without a chimney in which a fire is producing smoke at a constant rate. The room is ventilated with fresh air, but the rate of ventilation is adjustable. With ventilation set at some nominal level, the fresh air mixes with the smoke and the mixture is swept out of the window. If the ventilation of the room is halved, we might expect the smoke in the room to become twice as dense and we could describe the room as being hypercapnic (Greek *Kapnos* = smoke). Doubling the ventilation would halve the density of the smoke in the room. In each case the amount of smoke produced and pouring out of the window each minute is constant, but the smoke is mixed with a variable amount of air.

Suppose now that we keep the ventilation of the room constant but alter the rate of smoke production. It can easily be seen that doubling the rate would double the density of smoke in the room and double the rate at which smoke is emitted from the window. Halving the rate would halve density and emission.

We can summarize by saying that the density of smoke in the room depends upon the interplay of two factors:

1 Density *increases* as smoke production *increases*.
2 Density *increases* as ventilation *decreases*.

In the alveoli, a comparable condition exists. Carbon dioxide, produced in the tissues by metabolism, is carried to the lungs by the blood, and is poured out into the alveolar gas. The alveoli are ventilated by fresh air containing virtually no CO_2. The 'density' or concentration of CO_2 in alveolar gas thus depends, first, upon the rate at which CO_2 enters the alveoli (and this is set by the metabolic production of CO_2) and secondly upon the alveolar ventilation rate. But we have seen (p. 80) that in a gas mixture the partial pressure of any component gas is proportional to its concentration—as CO_2 concentration is doubled, alveolar P_{CO_2} is also doubled, and so on. We must therefore conclude that doubling CO_2 production without change in ventilation, or halving ventilation without change in CO_2 production, will double alveolar P_{CO_2}. If ventilation and CO_2 production are both doubled, alveolar P_{CO_2} will not change. This is what happens in health—alveolar ventilation keeps pace with the rate of production of CO_2.

It is now only necessary to point out that *the blood leaving the pulmonary capillaries (and thus the arterial blood) has a P_{CO_2} equal to that of the alveolar gas.* When we measure the P_{CO_2} of an arterial blood sample we are thus measuring, indirectly, alveolar P_{CO_2}. If this is normal it tells us that alveolar ventilation is adequate for the rate of production and elimination of CO_2. If arterial P_{CO_2} is abnormally high (more than 6 kPa or 45 mmHg, a condition termed *hypercapnia*) we can say that alveolar ventilation is too low, and the converse. Note that CO_2 is eliminated, over any extended period, as fast as it is produced, regardless of ventilation; the amount of smoke emitted from the window, in the example given above, depended on the rate at which the fire produced it, not upon the ventilation. The density of smoke was, however, affected by the ventilation of the room.

Ventilatory failure

When alveolar ventilation is persistently reduced to such an extent that the arterial P_{CO_2} is increased about 6 kPa (45 mmHg), ventilatory failure is said to be present. Following what has just been said about the factors which influence arterial P_{CO_2}, we may set down the following general causes of ventilatory failure.

1 *Reduction in alveolar ventilation* may occur in respiratory paralysis (due to disease of the nervous system or to large doses of muscle-relaxant drugs) or in depression of the respiratory centres (due to intracranial disease or overdosage with sedative or narcotic drugs).

2 *Inefficient alveolar ventilation.* Uneven matching of ventilation with blood flow (p. 77) leads to inefficiency, as though part of the alveolar ventilation were wasted. A normal alveolar ventilation may not be adequate under these conditions. If the patient is unable (because of weakness, oversedation or mechanical difficulties, p. 72) to produce the extra alveolar ventilation needed, ventilatory failure results. This is the situation commonly found in elderly, obese patients with chronic bronchitis, emphysema and acute respiratory infection.

3 *Increase in CO_2 production* is important in the postoperative period or in fever, when metabolism may be doubled. By itself this would not cause ventilatory failure, but it increases the demands made upon the ventilatory process and the patient may be unable to meet the demand.

The symptoms and signs of ventilatory failure, and its treatment, are described on pages 246 to 250.

Hypoxia

A patient with ventilatory failure, when breathing air, will not only have a high P_{CO_2} (hypercapnia) but in addition will suffer from lack of oxygen. Several terms are used to describe this state. *Anoxia* means 'without oxygen' and is never literally true in a living patient. *Hypoxia* means 'deficiency in oxygen' and is preferable. It may refer to hypoxic tissues or to a lowered PO_2 in arterial blood. *Hypoxaemia* refers specifically to blood and usually implies O_2 content rather than PO_2, but together with *asphyxia* (suffocation) it is better avoided altogether. In what follows hypoxia will mean a low PO_2 in arterial blood.

The lower limit of normal PO_2 in arterial blood is 11 kPa (85 mmHg), or 10 kPa (75 mmHg) in the elderly. Hypoxia may be caused by:

1   A reduced PO_2 in inspired air, as at high altitude. For example, in Mexico City (altitude 2270 m) inspired PO_2 is about 16 kPa (120 mmHg).

2   Underventilation of the alveoli as a whole; the hypoxia is always accompanied by a rise in arterial PCO_2.

3   Pulmonary disease with mismatching of ventilation and blood-flow in the alveoli; the hypoxia may be accompanied by a high, normal or even low arterial PCO_2, depending on the alveolar ventilation.

4   Anatomical defects allowing venous blood to be 'shunted' into the arterial side of the circulation; examples are atrial septal defect with reversal of flow, Fallot's tetralogy and complete obstruction of the airway (e.g. by carcinoma) of a region of lung which retains blood flow.

The recognition and treatment of hypoxia are described on p. 248 but some aspects of hypoxia and hypercapnia in ventilatory failure must be mentioned here.

Hypoxia and hypercapnia in ventilatory failure

If ventilatory failure is caused by drugs or paralysis, and the lungs are normal, correction of pulmonary ventilation will restore both PCO_2 and PO_2 in arterial blood to normal. On the other hand, if in addition the lungs are abnormal and ventilation and blood flow are mismatched, it is found that as ventilation is increased PCO_2 reaches normal levels before PO_2 is restored to normal—i.e. hypoxia persists even though hypercapnia is abolished. It may sometimes (but not always) be possible to abolish hypoxia by further increasing ventilation, but in this case PCO_2 will be lower than normal (hypocapnia). With mismatching of ventilation and blood flow (which is a very common defect in all pulmonary disease) it is not possible, while breathing ordinary air, to have a normal P_{CO_2} and normal P_{O_2} at the same time.

This dilemma is overcome as follows: If arterial P_{CO_2} is raised, the only way in which it can be lowered is to increase ventilation, if necessary by means of a respirator. Ventilation is adjusted until arterial P_{CO_2} is normal. If arterial P_{O_2} is still low, O_2 is added to increase arterial P_{O_2} to about 16 to 17 kPa (120 to 130 mmHg). This level ensures full O_2 saturation and allows a little margin in the case of mishap. It may be, of course, that high inspired O_2 (100 per cent O_2) is needed for some other reason (p. 85), but this is a separate problem.

5   The Kidneys

The kidneys perform three main functions:
1   They excrete many of the end-products of body metabolism.
2   They maintain water and electrolyte balance by varying excretion according to need.
3   They play a major part in the maintenance of acid-base balance.

Normal cellular function requires that the pH and the water and electrolyte content of the intracellular fluid (ICF, p. 9) be kept within narrow limits. This is achieved by the regulation of extracellular fluid (ECF) composition and by the special osmotic properties of the cell membrane (p. 8). In turn, the composition of ECF is very largely controlled by the kidneys. It is held almost constant in the face of wide fluctuations in the intake of food and water, and in metabolic activity. During the postoperative period, the kidneys are under increased stress at a time when renal function may be impaired.

Structure and function of the kidney

The general structure of the kidney is shown in Fig. 16. Each kidney is made up of about 1 million units called *nephrons*. A single nephron is illustrated in Fig. 17. Urine production starts at the glomerulus which filters fluid from blood. This fluid then passes along the tubular part of the nephron. During its passage its composition is modified and it emerges as urine from the collecting ducts into the renal pelvis.

The glomerulus (Fig. 17)

This is a tuft of capillaries almost surrounded by the glomerular capsule which leads into the proximal tubule. *The glomerulus allows*

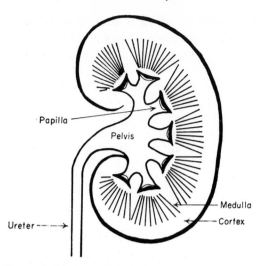

Papilla

Pelvis

Medulla

Cortex

Ureter

Fig. 16 General structure of the kidney.

a proportion of the capillary blood, minus cells and protein, to enter the capsule. The fluid entering the capsule is the *glomerular filtrate* which passes to the proximal tubule. The pressure in the glomerular capillaries is high (about 80 mmHg) and this forces fluid through the capillary and inner capsular walls and so into the tubular system. Red cells, and plasma proteins which have large molecules, remain in the circulation. About 1200 ml of blood flow through the glomeruli, and about 120 ml of filtrate pass into the glomerular capsule each minute (this is the *glomerular filtration rate*). The *creatinine clearance* gives a measure of the glomerular filtration rate. Two ml per sec amounts to 180 litres of glomerular filtrate each day. Since only 1·5 litres of urine are formed per day it is obvious that most of the filtrate (over 99 per cent) must be reabsorbed in its passage through the rest of the nephron.

Proximal tubule

In the proximal tubule much of the glomerular filtrate is reabsorbed and some substances are excreted. Almost all the potassium (K^+), and about 70 per cent of the sodium (Na^+), chloride (Cl^-), bicarbonate (HCO_3^-) and water are *reabsorbed* from the filtrate in the proximal tubule (Fig. 18). That is to say, these substances pass through the cells lining the tubule into the surrounding interstitial fluid and eventually into the tubular capillaries to rejoin the bloodstream. Many other substances (e.g. glucose, amino acids, uric acid) are also absorbed. Certain drugs, including penicillin, reach the urine by the opposite route; they are *excreted* from the tubular capillaries into the proximal tubular filtrate.

The total concentration of solute, i.e. dissolved particles (either ions or molecules, p. 5), does not change in the proximal tubule because solutes and water are reabsorbed in the same overall proportion in which they exist in plasma. Concentration or dilution is

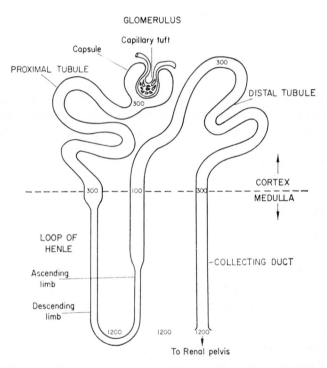

Fig. 17 Structure of a nephron. Figures in the tubule and interstitial region indicate the concentration (as 'osmolality') of the fluid in these situations. The high concentration in the interstitial fluid near the papillae and in the collecting duct (1200 mosm per l) is present when highly concentrated urine is being formed.

deferred until the more distal part of the nephron is reached. The concentration of the filtrate is measured as the number of dissolved particles of all kinds present in a litre of fluid; the units are milli-osmols per l (mosm per l). Representative concentrations in the nephron are shown in Fig. 17; the concentration of plasma is about 300 mosm per l.

Loop of Henle

The primary function of the loop of Henle is to produce a high osmolality in the interstitial fluid of the renal medulla. In the ascend-ing limb of the loop of Henle (Fig. 17) Na^+ and Cl^- are reabsorbed but the wall in this part of the loop is impermeable to water (Fig. 18). As a result the filtrate is diluted by the time it reaches the distal tubule. On the other hand the osmolality of the interstitial fluid rises because of the constant extrusion of Na^+ and Cl^- from the loop of Henle.

(Many of the particles producing the high osmolality in the inters-titial fluid are actually urea molecules, which follow Na^+ and Cl^- ions and become trapped in the interstitial fluid near the papillae). The high concentration of the interstitial fluid in the medulla is necessary for the proper functioning of the collecting ducts (see below), which pass through this region of the kidney.

Distal tubule

The main function of the distal tubule is the exchange of sodium passing down the tubule for potassium and hydrogen ions. It plays a major role in the regulation of acid-base balance. Most of the sodium filtered at the glomerulus, it will be remembered, is reabsorbed from the proximal tubule, and much of the rest from the ascending limb of the loop of Henle. About 25 000 mmol of sodium are filtered each day. Even the 1 or 2 per cent of this reaching the distal tubule is a critical amount in terms of sodium balance, since the normal daily intake of sodium is only 150 mmol. Consequently the final adjustments made by the distal tubule are of great importance.

The mechanism by which sodium is reabsorbed is under the control of *aldosterone* (p. 12). High secretion of this hormone favours Na^+ reabsorption in exchange for K^+, which is excreted into

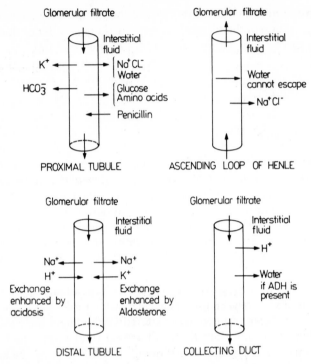

Fig. 18 Diagram to show the exchange of water, electrolytes and other products between various parts of the tubule and the nearby intestinal fluid (see text).

the distal tubule (Fig. 18). Absence of aldosterone (as in adrenal failure) promotes the excretion of Na^+ and the retention of K^+.

Alternatively, Na^+ may be reabsorbed in exchange for hydrogen ion (H^+) (Fig. 18). The extent to which this happens depends upon the availability of H^+, and is therefore increased in *acidosis*. The loss of H^+ from extracellular fluid reduces the acidosis. This is one way in which the kidneys help to regulate acid-base balance. The reabsorption of HCO_3^- in the proximal tubule obviously plays a major part in maintaining pH balance and is varied in the presence of respiratory or metabolic acidosis. The final adjustment made by the distal tubule is, however, important just as it is with sodium balance.

Apart from these actions, the distal tubules share to some extent in the concentrating function of the collecting ducts. This will now be described.

Collecting ducts

The collecting ducts regulate the amount of water excreted, and therefore urinary volume and concentration. The collecting ducts pass from the deeper part of the cortex through the renal medulla to the papillae. As a result of the action of the loops of Henle this is a region of high concentration. Osmotic forces (p. 8) therefore tend to cause water to pass out through the walls of the collecting ducts, thus concentrating their contents (Fig. 18). However, the wall of the collecting duct is only permeable to water if *antidiuretic hormone* (ADH, p. 12) is present in the blood. When water depletion has occurred, ADH is released into the blood by the

Table 8 Summary of renal function.

Site	Function	Mechanism
Glomerulus	Formation of glomerular filtrate (plasma minus its protein)	Simple filtration
Proximal tubule	*Reabsorption* into blood of (a) nearly all potassium (b) 70% of Na^+, Cl^-, HCO_3^-, and water (c) glucose, urea and other substances *Excretion* of penicillin	Special properties of tubular cells
Loop of Henle	Formation of concentrated fluid at the tip of the loop and in the surrounding medullary tissue	Complex process involving reabsorption of Na^+, and Cl^- from ascending limb of loop
Distal tubule	Exchange of Na^+ from tubular fluid for: (a) hydrogen ions and (b) potassium ions frm the blood	(a) depends on availability of hydrogen ions, i.e., on the acid-base state (b) enhanced by aldosterone
Collecting ducts	Reabsorption of water from tubular fluid to blood	Can occur only in the presence of anti-diuretic hormone (ADH)

pituitary gland, water is reabsorbed from the collecting duct, the urine is concentrated and water is conserved. On the other hand, if the body is well hydrated ADH disappears from the blood, water is not reabsorbed from the collecting duct, and a large volume of dilute urine is passed. Normal renal function is necessary for the proper operation of the ADH mechanism.

Other factors may bring about ADH release and water retention. ADH is released, for instance, in the postoperative period even if the patient is well hydrated. This effect is exaggerated if shock develops, or if certain drugs such as morphine or barbiturates are given.

Renal failure

The excretion by the kidney of unwanted metabolic end-products, and the selective retention of wanted substances, may be hindered in two general ways: (a) by reduction in glomerular filtration rate, and (b) by impairment of tubular function. As a rule these two functions are impaired together but occasionally impairment of one or other may predominate. Renal failure is best considered in relation to its cause.

Reduced blood-flow through the kidneys. When cardiac output is reduced, circulatory adjustments take place which help to direct the available flow to the organs which matter most for immediate survival — the heart and the brain. Since the kidneys normally take about $1/5$ of the cardiac output, a considerable saving is possible here. The mechanism is as follows: a fall in cardiac output reduces arterial blood pressure; via the baroreceptor reflex (p. 56) sympathetic activity is increased; the kidneys are particularly susceptible to vasoconstriction, and accordingly their vessels are powerfully narrowed.

As a result, renal blood-flow is reduced, and glomerular filtration rate diminishes. So little filtrate may reach the tubules that most or all of it is absorbed, and urine flow falls or even stops. There is an increase in plasma concentrations of urea, potassium and acids, and plasma pH falls. Phosphate rises and this causes a fall in ionized calcium. The rise in potassium and fall in ionized calcium concentrations increase myocardial irritability and dangerous arrhythmias may occur, especially in patients receiving digitalis preparations.

The excretion of digitalis, aminoglycoside antibiotics and many other drugs is diminished and the dose must be reduced.

When renal blood-flow is restored, filtration increases. If the renal ischaemia has lasted more than a few hours, *acute tubular necrosis* may result. In this case the phase of anuria or oliguria usually lasts several days and, when recovery begins, there is a phase of polyuria, due to the inability of the tubules to concentrate the filtrate. Electrolytes and water are lost excessively and have to be replaced. Unless tubular necrosis is extreme, recovery can occur in about 2 weeks.

Renal disease. In chronic pyelonephritis and chronic glomerulonephritis, nephrons are lost and replaced by scar tissue. Glomerular filtration and tubular activities are impaired. Renal disease is common in patients needing cardio-respiratory intensive care, and is important in that it reduces the renal reserve; consequently a fall in renal bloodflow, discussed above, is more damaging than in healthy kidneys.

6 Physiology of Cardiopulmonary Bypass

Techniques used in the operating room affect postoperative management and, although ICU staff are seldom involved in intra-operative management, an understanding of the techniques employed facilitates postoperative care.

CARDIOPULMONARY BYPASS

Most intracardiac operations are approached through a median sternotomy. The heart is exposed by incising the pericardium and cannulae are placed in the right atrium and the ascending aorta after administering heparin to prevent blood coagulation. The cannulae

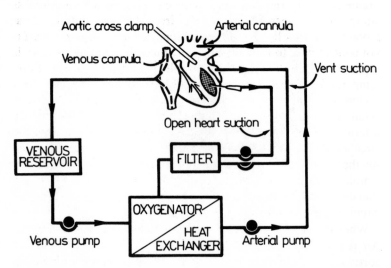

Fig. 19 Diagram of the extracorporeal circuit of the heart-lung machine.

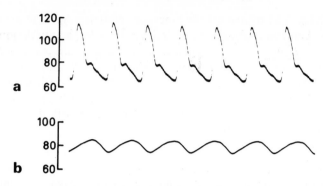

Fig. 20 Radial artery pressure tracings (mmHg). (a) Before cardiopulmonary bypass and (b) during cardiopulmonary bypass.

are connected to the extracorporeal circuit which has been primed with compatible blood or fluid from which air bubbles have been removed. This allows blood to be drained from the right atrium (or vena cavae), oxygenated, and returned via the aorta (Fig. 19).

As flow through the extracorporeal circuit is increased, blood is drained from the right atrium and the cardiac muscle fibres are less stretched. This decreases the output from the heart until the total blood flow is supplied by the heart/lung machine. Once the heart is not contributing to flow the normally pulsatile arterial pressure is replaced by a relatively non-pulsatile pressure (Fig. 20). Body temperature is reduced by cooling the blood with the heat exchanger. When the myocardium has been cooled, the aorta is clamped between the aortic cannulae and the origin of the coronary arteries, thus isolating the heart and the coronary system from the circulation (Fig. 19). It is clear that the extracorporeal circuit bypasses the heart and lungs and for this reason the lungs need not be ventilated during the period of cardiopulmonary bypass. Any blood that does enter the heart or pericardial cavity can be returned to the circuit via the vent or open heart suction (Fig. 19).

When the intracardiac repair is complete the patient is rewarmed. Air is carefully flushed from the chambers of the heart and the aortic cross-clamp is removed so that the coronary arteries are perfused again. The heart usually starts beating at this stage and, once it has fully recovered, the lungs are ventilated again. Drainage of blood into the extracorporeal circuit is slowed by manipulation of the venous reservoir (Fig. 19) and the atrial pressure is increased until the heart starts contributing to the flow. Cardiopulmonary bypass is then gradually discontinued until the total cardiac output is supplied by the heart. After the cannulae have been removed from the right atrium and aorta the action of heparin is reversed with protamine sulphate.

Prime of the extracorporeal circuit and haemodilution

Solutions used to prime the extracorporeal circuit vary from whole blood to those containing only 5 per cent dextrose in water. A common prime for adult patients consists of:

Lactated Ringer's solution	750–1000 ml
Dextrose 5 per cent in water	750–1000ml
Mannitol 15 per cent	300 ml
Total volume	1800–2300 ml

This prime volume represents about 30 to 40 per cent of the normal blood volume of an adult weighing 60 to 80 kg. It is clear that, when the prime and the patient's blood mix, the haemoglobin and serum protein concentrations are diluted to 70 to 80 per cent of the pre-bypass value. This dilution causes little problem provided the haemoglobin concentration does not fall below 70 to 80 g per litre (haematocrit 20 to 25 per cent). All the blood which remains in the extracorporeal circuit at the end of the operation is saved and retransfused into the patient. The excess fluid from the prime is excreted by the kidneys in the first few hours after the operation. This diuresis is accentuated by the osmotic effect of the mannitol in the prime and the hyperglycaemia associated with cardiopulmonary bypass.

The dilution is relatively larger in smaller patients, and the usual dilution would produce an unacceptably low haemoglobin concentration in patients who are anaemic preoperatively. For patients weighing less than 50 kg or with haemoglobin concentrations below 120 g per litre, a suitable priming solution is:

Citrated donor blood	1000 ml
Dextrose 4·3 per cent and	
NaCl 0·18 per cent in water	1000ml
Heparin	50 mg
KCl, CaCl₂, NAHCO₃	10 mmol each

A paediatric oxygenator primed with appropriately diluted citrated donor blood is used for children weighing less than 25 kg. Infants under 10 kg often undergo intracardiac surgery during profound hypothermia with circulatory arrest and for these operations the circuit is primed with fresh heparinized donor blood diluted if necessary to produce a postoperative haemoglobin concentration of 110 to 120 g per litre. When blood containing priming solutions is used it may not be necessary to retransfuse all the blood remaining in the oxygenator at the end of the procedure. Urine flow in the first few hours after the operation is often less than that seen with blood-free primes.

Haemodilution decreases oxygen delivery but this problem is overcome during cardiopulmonary bypass by the reduction of oxygen demand by hypothermia. In the paralysed patient, the oxygen requirement is reduced by 6 to 7 per cent for every degree the temperature is lowered. Haemodilution helps minimise damage to red blood corpuscles and platelets. Red cell damage leads to haemolysis and increased plasma haemoglobin which, if excessive, may cause renal failure, while platelet destruction is one of the causes of postoperative bleeding. The increase in plasma viscosity caused by hypothermia is offset by haemodilution but, if the dilution is excessive, osmotic pressure due to plasma proteins is decreased leading to oedema as fluid escapes from the capillaries.

Hypothermia

Some vascular beds become constricted during non-pulsatile perfusion. This is one of the reasons why perfusion during cardiopulmonary bypass is not as effective as natural perfusion. Suboptimal perfusion causes the moderate metabolic acidosis commonly found after cardiopulmonary bypass. Hypothermia reduces the effect of this poor perfusion by lowering the cellular oxygen demand. Oxygen consumption is 50 per cent of normal at 30°C, 25 per cent at 25°C, 15 per cent at 20°C and 10 per cent at 15°C. The low oxygen demand makes it possible to interrupt coronary perfusion for short periods during moderate hypothermia (25 to 30°C) or to stop the circulation for up to 1 hour at temperatures between 15 and 18°C. Profound hypothermia and circulatory arrest is often used for intracardiac surgery in infants under 10 kg. In this technique the patient is cooled to 15 to 18°C either by cold perfusion on cardiopulmonary bypass, or by surface cooling to about 25°C with final cooling on cardiopulmonary bypass. After hypothermic arrest rewarming is carried out by warm perfusion.

Hypothermia does not completely prevent the development of metabolic acidosis which may become apparent only after constricted vascular beds dilate again on rewarming. Some vascular beds remain constricted and cold at the end of rewarming bypass. As they dilate postoperatively, body temperature tends to fall again. Postoperative transfusion is required to fill the dilating vessels. Rewarming in the postoperative period may be accompanied by shivering which can increase the oxygen demand to 130 to 450 per cent of normal.

Myocardial protection

The aortic cross clamp (Fig. 19) isolates the coronary arteries from the circulation. During the period that the aorta is cross-clamped the myocardium can be protected either by decreasing its metabolic rate or by supplying the oxygen demand.

Cold cardioplegia decreases the metabolic rate by abolishing cardiac muscle activity and cooling the heart to 8 to 15°C. This is achieved by infusing a slightly hypotonic solution containing 20 to 30 mmol of potassium per litre at a temperature of 4°C through the coronary arteries. This allows the heart to remain unperfused for about 60 minutes and if more time is required, the cardioplegic infusion is repeated at 30 to 40 minute intervals. The infusion is also repeated if ECG activity recurs or if the myocardial temperature exceeds 20°C.

Intermittent release of the aortic cross-clamp. In this technique the aortic cross-clamp is released and the myocardium perfused for about 3 min every 20 to 30 min. This method can be used only when the aortic valve is intact and moderate hypothermia (25 to 30°C) is necessary to decrease myocardial oxygen demand during the cross-clamp periods.

Coronary perfusion supplies the oxygen demand. The coronary arteries are cannulated and perfused with oxygenated blood using two small pumps on the heart/lung machine. This perfusion is non-pulsatile. Coronary perfusion has been superseded by cold cardioplegia but is still occasionally used in patients with aortic incompetence.

2 Pharmacology

7 Drugs used in Intensive Care

Only the major groups of drugs are discussed here but reference to other drugs may be found in the index. Drugs are listed only by their approved name but common proprietary names can be found in Appendix 2.

DIURETICS

A diuretic is a substance which increases the excretion of water, or sodium and water, by the kidney, thus reducing the volume of the extra-cellular fluid (ECF). Diuretics may affect the proximal or the distal part of the nephron (pp. 90 to 96). For present purposes the *proximal* part of the nephron includes the proximal tubule, the loop of Henle and the beginning of the distal tubule, while the *distal* part of the nephron includes most of the distal tubule. Because the proximal nephron accounts for the greater part of sodium reabsorption, proximally-acting diuretics are more powerful; but distally-acting diuretics, which counteract the effects of aldosterone, are valuable when aldosterone levels are high. The most useful diuretics are:

Diuretics which act proximally
Osmotic diuretics: mannitol
Thiazides: chlorothiazide, cyclopenthiazide etc.
Frusemide (furosemide)

Diuretics which act distally
Spironolactone
Triamterene
Amiloride

107

Diuretics which act proximally

Osmotic diuretics. Mannitol passes into the glomerular capsule and, because of its osmotic effect (p. 8), it restricts the ability of the proximal tubule to reabsorb both water and sodium. A large volume of glomerular filtrate therefore reaches the distal nephron, swamping its capacity for reabsorption and producing a diuresis. If aldosterone levels are high, much of the sodium is reabsorbed in the distal tubule and dilute urine is produced. Mannitol causes a diuresis even when the patient is dehydrated. A high concentration of any particle in the blood will have the same effect. The diuresis which often occurs during and after cardiopulmonary bypass is partly due to the osmotic effects of high blood glucose and mannitol levels.

Thiazides and frusemide are nowadays the mainstay of diuretic treatment. These have their greatest effect in the loop of Henle. Reabsorption of sodium is inhibited and the maintenance of a highly concentrated interstitial fluid in the renal medulla is therefore impaired (p. 93). An extra load of sodium and water reaches the distal tubule and collecting duct, and diuresis results because reabsorption of water, which depends upon a high medullary interstitial concentration (p. 95), is reduced. Frusemide is more powerful and more rapidly acting than thiazides. Three other points should be noted:

1 Thiazides and frusemide present more sodium to the distal tubule. If aldosterone levels are high the exchange of potassium for sodium in the distal tubule may be greatly increased and heavy potassium loss may occur.

2 Thiazides and frusemide increase blood uric acid concentration and may precipitate gout.

3 They also tend to raise blood glucose concentration and may precipitate diabetes.

Diuretics which act distally

The action of aldosterone on the distal tubules is blocked by spironolactone. The exchange of potassium for sodium is inhibited, with the result that potassium is conserved and more sodium is excreted. Although spironolactone is much less powerful than the proximally-acting diuretics it can be very effective when used in conjunction with them. When proximally-acting diuretics are administered in the presence of high aldosterone levels a great deal of potassium is exchanged for sodium in the distal tubules (see above). This limits the excretion of sodium and increases the loss of potassium. The addition of spironolactone can overcome these problems although it has to be administered for two or three days before it becomes effective. Two other drugs with a similar effect (produced by a different mechanism) are amiloride and triamterene. These drugs provide a useful alternative to potassium supplements, but hyperkalaemia may occur in the presence of impaired renal function.

DRUGS ACTING ON THE CARDIOVASCULAR SYSTEM

The effects of many drugs on the cardiovascular system cannot be described without reference to the electrocardiogram and to various abnormal rhythms. These are dealt with in chapter 8, which should be read in conjunction with the following account.

Digoxin

Actions

1 Increases cardiac *contractility*, i.e. the speed and force of contraction.
2 Increases cardiac *irritability*, i.e. the tendency to develop ectopic beats. These, particularly when alternating with normal sinus beats, are a common sign of excessive dosage.
3 Slows *conduction* of the cardiac impulse and increases the P–R interval; in excessive dosage digoxin can thus cause heart block.
4 Slows *recovery of the A–V node* (p. 42) after each beat. The node thus responds to fewer impulses from the atria in atrial fibrillation, and the ventricular rate is reduced.
5 By controlling cardiac failure digoxin has many secondary effects, e.g. diuresis and the reduction of heart rate and venous pressure.

Uses

1 Control of cardiac failure with or without arrhythmias.

2 Control of certain arrhythmias with or without cardiac failure, particularly atrial fibrillation and supraventricular tachycardia.

Dosage

'Digitalizing' dose. 1 to 2 mg orally, 0·5 to 1·5 mg intravenously, in divided doses spread over 1 to 2 days. For infants under 2 years old, a maximum of 70 μg per kg (70 μg = 0·07 mg). Over 2 years of age, the dose is 50 μg per kg (the adult dose works out at about 40 μg per kg).

Maintenance dose. 0·25 to 0·75 mg daily, orally. Under 2 years of age, 10 to 20 μg per kg daily and over 2 years 10 μg per kg daily, in divided doses orally (see also p. 285).

Toxic effects

1 Loss of appetite, nausea and vomiting, usually in that order.
2 Almost any arrhythmia can be caused by digoxin. Ventricular extrasystoles (premature beats) are the commonest and often alternate with sinus beats. Ventricular tachycardia and fibrillation, supraventricular tachycardia and atrial fibrillation also occur.
3 Sinus bradycardia may be the only feature in infants, and digoxin may have to be withheld if the rate falls below 60 per min.
4 Atrioventricular block (A–V block).

Toxic effects occur more readily when body potassium is depleted; the serum potassium need not be low, but sometimes is. Digoxin is largely excreted in the urine, and in renal failure only half the usual dose may be needed. Digoxin must be stopped at once if toxicity arises; potassium may be needed, orally or intravenously at up to 20 mmol per hour. Calcium aggravates digitalis poisoning and its intravenous administration may cause sudden death. Antiarrhythmic drugs (see below) may be needed in digitalis-induced arrhythmias. Serum levels of digoxin are a useful aid in deciding whether an arrhythmia is due to digitalis toxicity or not. In the absence of potassium depletion, toxic effects are uncommon if the serum digoxin concentration is less than 2·5 μmol per l (2 ng per ml), but become increasingly common when the concentration rises above 3 μmol per l (2·5 ng per ml). Toxic effects are less common in infants who usually tolerate levels of 4 μmol per l (3 ng per ml).

Drugs used in the treatment of arrhythmias

The use of digoxin has already been described. Other drugs commonly used in the treatment of arrhythmias can be conveniently arranged in four groups.

Group 1. Quinidine-like drugs. Quinidine, procainamide, lignocaine, mexilitine, disopyramide, phenytoin.

Group 2. Beta adrenergic blockers. Propranolol.

Group 3. Drugs which prolong the action potential. Amiodarone.

Group 4. Drugs which block entry of calcium into the myocardial cell. Verapamil, perhexiline.

Drugs within each group show some variation and there is overlap of properties between the groups, but the classification forms a useful framework on which to build an understanding of the drug therapy of arrhythmias.

Group 1. Quinidine-like drugs

Actions

1 All these drugs diminish myocardial *excitability* and thus suppress beats which arise from foci other than the normal pacemaker.

2 All decrease myocardial *contractility* to some extent and thus reduce cardiac output and blood pressure in large doses or in sensitive patients.

3 Quinidine, procainamide and mexilitine depress *conduction* of the cardiac excitation wave.

Uses

1 *Ventricular tachycardia.* Lignocaine is usually the first choice, followed by procainamide or mexilitine. In the dose usually required, quinidine is more toxic than the other drugs.

2 *Ventricular extrasystoles*

a Occurring after myocardial infarction or cardiac surgery, frequent ventricular extrasystoles often herald the more serious ventricular tachycardia. Their treatment is the same.

b As an isolated feature, frequent enough to cause palpitation but not thought to presage ventricular tachycardia, extrasystoles provide the main indication nowadays for quinidine.

3 *Supraventricular extrasystoles and tachycardia.* Intravenous

Table 9 Anti-arrhythmia drugs.

Drug	Toxic effects	Dosage
Quinidine	1 Allergic reactions (rashes, oedema, collapse, acute asthma, purpura) 2 Tinnitus, headache, nausea 3 Heart block, cardiac arrest	Test dose 200 mg orally. 200–300 mg 4–6-hourly orally. 10 mg per min IV. Smaller doses needed in renal failure
Procainamide	Allergic reactions as for quinidine 2 Heart block, cardiac arrest 3 A syndrome resembling lupus erythematosus, with prolonged use	250–500 mg 6-hourly orally (sometimes even 1 g 4-hourly). 50 mg per min IV. Smaller doses needed in renal failure
Lignocaine (Lidocaine)	1 Drowsiness, coma, convulsions 2 Hypotension	IV only, 1–2 mg per kg given over 30 sec, followed by 1–3 mg per min by continuous infusion. A single dose acts for 10–20 min
Mexilitine	1 Nausea, vomiting, bad taste 2 Blurred vision, confusion 3 Hypotension, bradycardia	100–250 mg IV in 10 minutes, 250 mg in 1 hr, 250 mg in 2 hr, then 0·5–1 mg per min. Orally 200–250 mg 3–4 times daily
Disopyramide	1 Anticholinergic — dry mouth, blurred vision, hesitancy of micturition, gastrointestinal upset 2 Heart block, heart failure, cardiac arrest	3 mg per kg IV over 1 hr, then 0·4 mg per kg per hr. Maintenance 400–600 mg daily by mouth
Phenytoin	1 Asystole if injected quickly 2 Tremors, ataxia, diplopia, headache 3 Skin rash, anaemia 4 Overgrowth of gums	4 mg per kg IV over 5 min. Maintenance 200–400 mg daily by mouth

Note: ECG and blood pressure should be monitored whenever these drugs are given intravenously.

disopyramide is useful in suppressing supraventricular ectopics which may progress to supraventricular tachycardia or atrial fibrillation if untreated; if oral treatment is feasible, quinidine is the alternative.

It should be emphasised that cardioversion (p. 115) is usually more effective for tachy arrhythmias than any of these drugs.

Toxic effects and dosage (Table 9)

Where maximal dosage is needed to achieve the desired therapeutic effect, or where toxicity is suspected, serum levels of these drugs should be measured. There is usually a peak about 1 hour after an oral dose, but the level just before the next dose is a more useful guide (Table 10). Unless an initial loading dose is given, a stable serum level may not be achieved for 2 or 3 days.

Table 10 Blood levels of anti-arrhythmia drugs.

Drug	Therapeutic level (serum)		Level at which toxic symptoms become common	
	μg/ml	μmol/l	μg/ml	μmol/l
Quinidine	2–6	6–18	9	28
Procainamide	4–8	15–30	12	45
Lignocaine	2–6	9–26	10	43
Mexilitine	0·5–2	3–11	3	16
Disopyramide	3–6	9–18	7	20
Phenytoin	10–15	40–60	20	80

Group 2. Beta adrenergic blocking drugs

Propranolol (see also p. 33).

Actions

By blocking beta adrenergic receptors, propranolol helps to suppress ectopic ventricular foci. At the same time both heart rate and conduction are slowed, and contractility is impaired; if the heart is dependent upon sympathetic stimuli, cardiac failure may be precipitated.

Uses

1 Suppression of ventricular arrhythmias including those due to digitalis.
2 Less effectively, in supraventricular arrhythmias.
3 For the long-term treatment of angina of effort and of hypertension.
4 For temporary control of cyanotic spells in tetralogy of Fallot.

Dosage

Orally: 10 to 80 mg 4 times daily. Long-acting preparations are available.
Intravenously: 1 mg per min to a total of 5 mg.

Toxic effects

1 Dizziness, nausea, vomiting and diarrhoea.
2 Hypotension, bradycardia, cardiac failure.
3 Hypoglycaemia.
4 Bronchoconstriction which is dangerous in asthmatic patients.
    There are many beta-receptor blocking drugs which differ from propranolol in specific ways. For example, *oxprenolol, alprenolol* and *pindolol* have a slight *intrinsic inotropic effect* (separate from their beta-blocking effect), whereas propranolol has a slight intrinsic depressant action. Cardioselective beta blockers have little effect on the beta receptors in the bronchial wall and peripheral vessels. For practical purposes, however, there is little to choose between individual beta-receptor blocking drugs in the management of arrhythmias.

Group 3. Drugs which prolong the action potential

Amiodarone has proved an extremely effective drug for the control of both supraventricular and ventricular arrhythmias, often when other drugs have failed. It is given orally in dosages varying from 200 to 1200 mg daily and it may take a week or more to demonstrate its full effect. Fatigue and hypersensitivity to the sun are its most common side effects and long-term effects have yet to be established. Because of the slow onset of action it plays little role in the ICU.

Group 4. Calcium antagonists

Verapamil is the most effective drug for interrupting a supraventricular tachycardia. Up to 5 mg is given intravenously over 1 to 2 minutes, repeated if required in 10 minutes. A–V block and severe hypotension may occur if the injection is too rapid.

Other treatment of arrhythmias

1 *Pressure on eyeballs or carotid sinuses* causes vagal stimulation (p. 30) and may stop a supraventricular tachycardia.

2 *Edrophonium,* a short-acting anticholinesterase (p. 33) magnifies the effect of carotid sinus pressure by delaying the destruction of ACh at cardiac vagal endings.

3 *Antihistamine drugs* are sometimes effective in treating supraventricular tachycardia.

4 *Cardioversion* ('DC shock') is most conveniently described in full here. It consists in the brief application of a direct current of electricity to the heart, either directly at operation or indirectly through the chest wall. The current depolarizes the whole heart, including the ectopic focus or foci, and the sequence of abnormal activation is broken. Usually the sinus node is the first region to recover and sinus rhythm is often restored. There is, however, one important qualification. If DC shock coincides with the T wave of the ECG in either supraventricular tachycardia or atrial fibrillation, it may cause ventricular fibrillation. In these arrhythmias it is thus necessary to synchronize the shock with the 'safe' period of the cardiac cycle, and by a special ECG linkage the shock is timed to coincide with the QRS complex. In ventricular tachycardia synchronization is not necessary and in ventricular fibrillation it is not possible. If successful, DC shock restores sinus rhythm within 30 sec, often after a few bizarre complexes have occurred.

Uses. Cardioversion is the most effective way of restoring sinus rhythm in *supraventricular tachycardia, atrial fibrillation and atrial flutter.* It is the only effective treatment in *ventricular fibrillation* (though alternating current shock is almost as good) and in many cases of *ventricular tachycardia.*

Premedication. In a fully digitalised patient cardioversion will occasionally cause intractable ventricular fibrillation, despite shock

synchronization; digitalis should therefore be stopped 48 hours
before the procedure. Where feasible quinidine or disopyramide is
started the day before cardioversion is carried out. When ventricular arrhythmias prove resistant to DC shock, the administration
of propranolol may allow cardioversion to succeed. If the arrhythmia has been present for more than 2 weeks, a period of 3 to 4 weeks
anticoagulation precedes cardioversion to minimise the risk of
embolism.

Technique of cardioversion. The electrodes are placed either one in
front and one behind the chest, or one is applied to the right of the
upper sternum and the other over the cardiac apex. A liberal coat of
electrode paste on the electrodes and firm application of these to
the chest wall ensure good transmission of the depolarizing current
to the heart and avoid burning the skin. Electrode paste can be
replaced by commercially available electrode strips. For *supraventricular arrhythmias* the control is switched to the 'cardioversion'
position and the oscilloscope is checked to ensure that the cardioversion (synchronised) artefact falls on the QRS complex. For
ventricular arrhythmias the control is switched to the 'defibrillation'
position and no artefact is seen on the oscilloscope trace. The
appropriate energy output is selected, the machine is charged and
cardioversion is then attempted. The energy level is measured in
joules (J), also known as watt-seconds (Ws); 5 to 10 may be enough
for an infant but an adult may need 50 to 300 J. It is best to start with
the lower energy output and, if necessary, increase to higher levels
for subsequent attempts.

Cardioversion may damage an artificial pacemaker. An external
pacemaker should therefore be disconnected before the procedure,
and in patients with an implanted pacemaker cardioversion should
be avoided if at all possible. Older ECG machines may also be
damaged if connected during cardioversion, and unless you are sure
your machine has built-in protection (as have most modern instruments) it is best to unplug the patient cable beforehand.

Sympathomimetic drugs

These have been discussed in detail in Chapter 2 (Autonomic
nervous system) and are dealt with later in Chapter 9 (Cardiac
intensive care). It is necessary here only to summarize the indica-

tions for and dosage of the most important cardiovascular sympa-thomimetic drugs.

Isoprenaline (Isoproterenol)

Uses

1 To improve A–V conduction in heart block of first or second degree.
2 To increase ventricular rate in complete heart block.
3 To increase the force of ventricular contraction.
   The effect of these actions is to increase an inadequate cardiac output.

Dosage

1 By intravenous infusion. Up to 0·5 μg per kg per min, prefer-ably, for accuracy, from a constant infusion pump; most patients respond, if at all, to a quarter of this dose.
2 By mouth, as 'Saventrine' (a long-acting form of isoprenaline) 15 to 90 mg 6-hourly.
3 Sublingually or rectally, 5 to 10 mg 2-hourly.

Toxic effects

Tremor and anxiety often occur and may diminish with sedation. Sinus tachycardia is very common and the rate may limit the dosage possible. Sometimes the rate will slow if a further volume load is given. Ventricular extrasystoles are often the first sign that a safe dose of isoprenaline has been exceeded; if the dose is not reduced, ventricular tachycardia and fibrillation may ensue. Careful monitor-ing of the ECG is essential during the infusion of isoprenaline.

Dopamine and dobutamine

Uses

These drugs are used for their inotropic action, increasing the speed and strength of ventricular contraction with little effect on heart rate.

Dosage

Dosage range varies from 2·5 to 50 μg per kg per min but the usual effective range is 4 to 10 μg per kg per min; if this dosage is not effective additional measures are usually required.

Toxic effects

Toxic effects are the same as with isoprenaline but side effects are usually minor with moderate dosage.

Adrenaline (Epinephrine)

Uses

The administration of adrenaline, as distinct from isoprenaline, is usually limited to the treatment of acute circulatory collapse (p. 202) including severe allergic reactions.

Dosage

1   100 μg (1 ml of 1/10 000 solution) IV, repeated as necessary.
2   By continuous intravenous infusion, at the same rate as for isoprenaline.

Vasodilator drugs

In the ICU vasodilator drugs may be required for control of hypertension or, more commonly, to lower the work load of the heart. Many drugs are now available (Table 11). In using them certain principles must be borne constantly in mind.

1   A given agent may preferentially dilate arterioles and therefore be used primarily to reduce the *afterload* against which the heart must work (effectively the systemic vascular resistance), or it may preferentially dilate the venous bed and so reduce the *preload* (the left ventricular end-diastolic pressure). Phentolamine and hydralazine dilate arterioles, nitrates dilate veins, and nitroprusside dilates both.

2   Other factors affect the response of the vascular bed, the most important being hypoxia and acidosis. The aim of arteriolar dilata-

Table 11 Vasodilator drugs in common use.

Direct vasodilators	Nitroprusside, nitrates, hydralazine, diazoxide, nitroglycerine
Alpha receptor blockers	Prazosin, labetalol, (also beta), phentolamine, phenoxybenzamine
Beta receptor stimulants	Isoprenaline
Sympathetic ganglion or neurone blockers	Trimetaphan, guanethidine, reserpine
Angiotensin—2 inhibitors	Captopril
Calcium antagonists	Verapamil, nifedipine, perhexiline
Centrally acting (brain)	Clonidine, methyldopa
Diuretics	Frusemide

tion is to improve peripheral perfusion. This will improve blood gases, and thereby improve cardiac output, so that a new equilibrium may be established with better flows but without much change in blood pressure (remember BP = CO × SVR, p. 50). Venous dilatation will reduce pulmonary capillary pressure, improve respiratory function and blood gases, and reduce dyspnoea.

Other drugs may affect the response. For example, if a hypotensive agent has been given preoperatively and is not completely excreted, the response to a vasodilator agent may be unexpectedly brisk.

3 A sudden fall in blood pressure must be avoided. Strict monitoring is required and drugs with rapid action and rapid metabolism are preferred to longer-acting drugs, so that precise dosage can be titrated according to response.

Details of the drugs most commonly used intravenously are given in Table 12. For the *treatment of hypertension* the most rapid response is obtained with sodium nitroprusside. Alternatives are intravenous hydralazine or clonidine. Labetalol (2 mg per min to a maximum of 200 mg) is sometimes used but the beta-blocking component of this drug makes it unsuitable if heart failure is present. If additional treatment is required frusemide, IM reserpine (0·1

Table 12 Vasodilator drugs used in the ICU.

Drug	Dosage	Preload reduction	Afterload reduction	Side effects
Nitroprusside	IV 0·5–4 μg/kg/min, rarely 10 μg/kg/min	+++	+++	Hypotension, vomiting, lactic acidosis (cyanide), neurological symptoms (thiocyanate)
Nitroglycerine	IV 0·5–2 μg/kg/min, rarely 4 μg/kg/min	+++	+	Hypotension, vomiting, headache, flushing
Phentolamine	IV 2–30 μg/kg/min	+	+++	Hypotension, vomiting, headache, tachycardia
Hydralazine	IV 0·05–0·3 mg/kg repeat 4–6 hourly	0	++	Hypotension, vomiting, headache, tachycardia
Clonidine	IV 2 μg/kg in 10 min, repeat once if required and 6-hourly			Transient hypertension, hypotension, neurological symptoms

to 0·5 mg per dose) or a beta blocker may be used. For continued treatment the patient will be changed to oral medication. Depending on the difficulty of control this may include a diuretic, a beta blocker, and a vasodilator such as prazosin.

In the *treatment of low cardiac output* phentolamine or hydralazine are sometimes favoured if pure afterload reduction is required. Both may produce a tachycardia and many units prefer sodium nitroprusside. Sodium nitroprusside is converted by red cells to cyanmethaemoglobin and free cyanide; the cyanide is then converted by the liver to thiocyanate which in turn is cleared very slowly by the kidneys. Sodium nitroprusside must be protected from light. Rapid administration may cause cyanide accumulation producing lactic acidosis. With renal impairment thiocyanate will accumulate producing tinnitus, blurred vision and delirium. With prolonged treatment it is necessary to check blood gases to ensure there is no metabolic acidosis. Thiocyanate levels are also measured, the toxic level being 100 μg per ml or 1·7 mmol/l. For long-term management oral treatment with hydralazine, prazosin, nifedipine or captopril may be maintained.

Nitroglycerine is the treatment of choice for the reduction of preload. For prolonged treatment isosorbide dinitrate or nitroglycerine paste are usually the most convenient ways to administer nitrates.

In practice, vasodilators are almost always given in the ICU with inotropic agents. Combined use of these drugs is discussed further in Chapter 9.

INFECTION AND ANTIBIOTICS

Bacterial or viral infection is the result of an interaction between the invading organism and the tissues of the patient—the 'seed' and the 'soil'. An assault by bacteria or viruses does not necessarily cause infection. The outcome depends upon the state of the patient's natural defences on the one hand, and the capacity of the organism to overcome them (*pathogenicity*) and its invasiveness (*virulence*) on the other. The number of invading organisms is also a factor.

The natural defences

Structural. The skin and membranes lining the bronchi, alimentary tract and urinary system form barriers to the spread of micro-organisms. Each has special qualities, e.g. the ciliary processes of the bronchial lining (p. 68). These surfaces all produce secretions which have a protective function. If these secretions are dried up either by the action of drugs or artificial ventilation then the surface becomes more liable to infection.

Cellular. Certain cells, widely distributed in blood and tissues are able to ingest and kill bacteria. The most familiar are the neutrophil leucocytes of blood (polymorphonuclear cells), which increase in number in many bacterial infections but usually not in viral infections. These cells accumulate in areas of infection to form abscesses.

Other cells, the lymphocytes, multiply in lymph nodes which drain an infected area, and the nodes become enlarged. Lymphocytes in nodes and spleen are mainly responsible for the manufacture of antibodies.

Chemical. Substances called *antibodies* are produced in response to many infections and have the property of destroying the specific organism concerned. Sometimes they persist throughout life but more often they gradually disappear unless 'boosted' by reinfection or artificial inoculation. They are the main defence against viruses. The body also possesses certain antibodies which are not specific to one type of organism and which are present throughout life. Antibodies are proteins called *gammaglobulins.* Rarely, a patient is congenitally unable to produce gammaglobulins and is an easy prey to infection.

These defences are weakened by prolonged or debilitating illness and by malnutrition. They are poorly developed in young infants and gradually decline in old age.

A good example of the importance of the 'soil' in infection is the development of bacterial endocarditis. This is commonly due to *Streptococcus viridans,* a common organism of rather low pathogenicity and virulence which is often released from the roots of teeth into the bloodstream at the time of dental extractions or even in the act of chewing. This *bacteraemia* is normally short-lived and unnoticed. However, in the presence of rheumatic heart disease, the bacteria may settle in the damaged valves, multiply there and produce intermittent showers of organisms in the blood; this is *septicaemia*, because infection is established, and the streptococcus may be cultured repeatedly from the blood. The occurrence of infection is due to a breach in the structural defences, namely the damaged valve. Artifical valves are also prone to infection.

The invading organism

Since for practical purposes there is no treatment for viral infections, the rest of this account will be concerned mainly with bacteria.

Bacteria vary greatly in pathogenicity and virulence. Many are able to survive in the mouth, skin and colon without invading these tissues. Occasionally, as in the case of *Streptococcus viridans*, a lowering of the defences enables such a bacterium to infect. Others are equally widespread but require special conditions to cause infection; for example, *Clostridium tetani*, the cause of tetanus, is found everywhere in humus and soil, but cannot multiply until it is implanted in a wound beneath the skin and largely excluded from oxygen. Yet others, e.g. *Streptococcus pneumoniae* ('pneumococcus') or *Salmonella typhi*, are capable of infecting apparently healthy people through intact membranes. Bacteria must be able to attach themselves to mucosal surfaces to produce this type of infection. Sometimes the invasion of tissues by an organism is favoured by an alteration in the customary balance of bacteria, e.g. the yeast *Candida albicans* may flourish unchallenged when alimentary bacteria are suppressed by wide-spectrum antibiotics, and *Pseudomonas pyocyanea* tends to flourish in wounds from which other bacteria have been eliminated.

The identification of bacteria

When a bacterium is isolated from an infected area, or from an area at risk of infection, its identification gives a most valuable guide as to the likely course of infection and the type of antibiotic most likely to be effective in treatment. Bacteria are classified by the following features:

1 *Staining reaction under the microscope.* Gram's stain is the most useful; bacteria staining blue are 'Gram-positive' and red 'Gram-negative'. Several special staining methods are used, e.g. the Ziehl-Nielson method for tubercle bacilli, which keep their stain even when exposed to dilute acid (hence 'acid-fast' bacilli).

2 *Microscopic appearance.* The main forms are rods (*bacilli*) and spheres (*cocci*). Cocci grouped in chains are called *streptococci* and in clumps *staphylococci*. Motility is another characteristic which helps to identify bacteria, e.g. *E. coli, Klebsiella.*

3 *Cultural behaviour*, e.g. the ability to ferment various sugars, helps in the finer classification of bacteria. Sometimes the naked-eye appearance of the culture-plate is characteristic, e.g. the yellow colonies of *Staphylococcus aureus.*

4 *Immunological methods.* Prepared antibodies are added to bacterial cultures and their effect noted.

Table 13 lists the more important bacteria according to Gram's stain and microscopic appearance, together with the antibiotics to which they are most often sensitive.

Infection in the intensive care unit

A patient in the ICU is particularly susceptible to infection since he is already seriously ill and his defences are impaired (p. 121). He runs an important risk of *cross-infection,* which is transmitted in several ways:

1   From respirators, humidifers and incubators, which should be sterilized regularly and always when transferred from one patient to another. Intravenous infusion sets should be changed every 48 hr for the same reason.

2   From the attendant's hands. Scrupulous washing of the hands should be carried out before attention to dressings, catheters, etc., and sterile gloves should be used for tracheal aspiration.

3   From the nose and throat of the attendants. *Staphylococcus aureus* (nose) and *Streptococcus pyogenes* (throat) are likely to be transmitted in this way.

4   From airborne dust particles, bedding, clothing, etc. Culture of the dust in an ICU closely reflects the bacteriological climate of the ward, even to the antibiotic resistances of the bacteria concerned. The emergence of resistant strains of bacteria during treatment is thus a risk not only to the patient being treated but to all the other patients exposed to cross-infection. Frequent cleaning of walls and floors with antiseptic solutions, good ventilation of the ICU, and meticulous cleaning of all instruments and ward furniture go far to minimize the constant threat of cross-infection.

The portal of entry of infection may be the surgical wound, intravascular catheterization sites, a catheterized bladder, an intubated trachea, a tracheostomy wound or broken skin over pressure areas. The mere presence of bacteria in any of these sites does not necessarily indicate infection; other features (redness, suppuration, fever, leucocytosis) should be looked for before deciding to treat the patient with an antibiotic. In general, the use of an antibiotic to *prevent* cross-infection is bad practice and ultimately results in widespread bacterial resistance to the antibiotics used.

Antibiotics

Antibiotics are substances produced by a wide range of moulds, which suppress or kill many pathogenic bacteria without unduly harming the patient. Some antibiotics are *bacteristatic*, i.e. they stop the bacteria multiplying but do not kill them; the final elimination of

Table 13 Common pathogenic bacteria.

Organism	Probable sensitivity
Cocci	
1 Gram-positive	
Staphylococcus aureus	CLX, CLD, CPD
Streptococcus pyogenes	BP, A, CTM
S. viridans	BP, G
S. faecalis	A, G
S. pneumoniae	BP, A
2 Gram-negative	
Neisseria meningitidis	BP, A, CRC
Bacilli	
1 Gram-positive	
Clostridium welchii	BP, A, M, CLD
Cl. tetani	BP, A, M, CLD
2 Gram-negative	
Haemophilus influenzae	A, CRC
Escherichia coli	A, G, CFX, Tt
Klebsiella pneumoniae	G, CFX, CTM
K. aerogenes	G, CFX, Tt
Proteus mirabilis	G, CFX, Tt
P. vulgaris	G, CFX
Salmonella (various)	A, CFX
Pseudomonas pyocyanea	G, Tc
Bacteroides	M, CLD, CXT
Yeasts	
Candida albicans	Amphotericin B
	5-fluorocytosine

Symbols

A	ampicillin	CTM	cotrimoxazole
BP	benzylpenicillin	CXT	cefoxitin
CFX	cefuroxine	G	gentamicin
CLD	clindamycin	M	metronidazole
CPD	cephradine	Tc	ticarcillin
CRC	chloramphenicol	Tt	tetracycline

bacteria is left to the natural defences. Others are *bactericidal*, and kill the bacteria if given in adequate doses. In general, these properties are as listed on page 126.

Bactericidal	**Bacteristatic**
Benzylpenicillin	Chloramphenicol
Cloxacillin	Tetracycline
Ampicillin	Erythromycin
Amoxycillin	Co-trimoxazole
Cephradine	
Streptomycin	
Amikacin	
Gentamicin	

In the critical situation so often present in the ICU, bactericidal antibiotics are preferred to bacteristatic ones.

Selection of an antibiotic

Identification of the bacteria (p. 122). Sometimes this is enough; for example, all strains of *S. pyogenes* are sensitive to benzylpenicillin. At other times, an intelligent guess can be made; e.g. *S. viridans* is likely to succumb to a combination of benzylpenicillin and gentamicin. Likely sensitivities of other bacteria are shown in Table 13. If a patient is very ill a start can be made with the most likely antibiotic until the sensitivity tests are reported, and a change then made if necessary.

Sensitivity tests to antibiotics. The effect of various concentrations of different antibiotics can be observed in cultures of the bacterium concerned. The one which suppresses the organism in the lowest concentration will probably be the antibiotic of choice, but a bactericidal one takes precedence over a bacteristatic one. The demonstration of sensitivity in culture does not guarantee clinical effectiveness, although a culturally less active antibiotic should only be given after careful deliberation.

Known behaviour of organism. Experience has shown that the sensitivities of some bacteria may change during treatment; this occurs, for example, with rifamycin and nalidixic acid. The development of resistance to rifamycin can be prevented if it is used in combination with another antibiotic such as vancomycin. This combination is sometimes used to treat difficult cases of endocarditis.

Previous reactions of the patient, and known toxic actions of the antibiotic. A previous reaction such as a skin rash should lead to the choice of another antibiotic; patients or their relatives should always be questioned about previous antibiotic therapy. Antibiotics of known toxicity, e.g. chloramphenicol and gentamicin are avoided when a less toxic one would serve.

Reactions to antibiotics

All antibiotics carry some risk to the patient, because of either a particular sensitivity of the patient or a general toxic property of the antibiotic.

1 *Hypersensitivity reactions* consist of fever, malaise and an urticarial rash, or a profound anaphylactic shock, often fatal. Unfortunately there is no certain way of predicting the more serious of these unless the patient has survived a previous episode of the same kind. Penicillin is the main offender. Severe anaphylaxis is treated with adrenaline and steroid.

2 *Toxic effects.* All antibiotics are potentially toxic. Thus streptomycin and gentamicin can cause deafness; they, amikacin and amphotericin can cause renal damage, chloramphenicol can damage the bone marrow and the tetracyclines can give rise to severe gastrointestinal upsets. Penicillin can cause a fatal epileptiform fit if high doses are given to a patient in renal failure. With most antibiotics it is important to check renal function regularly because renal impairment, due either to the action of the antibiotic itself or to some other cause, may lead to high blood levels of the antibiotic with severe toxic reactions.

3 *Superinfection* occurs when a resistant organism 'fills the vacuum' created when a wide-spectrum antibiotic eliminates the natural bacterial population.

Bacterial resistance to antibiotics

An antibiotic may fail to suppress or kill an organism because the organism is merely indifferent to its presence (the usual reason) or because the organism actually destroys the antibiotic (seen in penicillin-resistant staphylococci). A culture of bacteria predominantly sensitive to an antibiotic may contain a few organisms which are resistant. The antibiotic eliminates the sensitive ones and the resistant strain multiplies. This may happen in a patient infected with staphylococci. Even when the organism is reported as sensitive to penicillin, the presence of an unrecognized strain may become apparent during treatment. The resistant strains produce an enzyme, penicillinase, which destroys benzylpenicillin. Cloxacillin is a penicillin which is not inactivated by penicillinase.

Antibiotic-resistance is a considerable practical problem, and sensitivity tests should be repeated during treatment to make sure that the organism is still sensitive to the antibiotic being used. Combinations of antibiotics are sometimes used to avoid or deter the emergence of resistant strains, on the grounds that a bacterial variant is unlikely to be resistant to two unrelated antibiotics.

Conclusions

A detailed account of individual antibiotics is beyond the aims of this book, but the following principles deserve emphasis.

1 Whenever possible the organism must be identified and its sensitivities determined before treatment begins, and at intervals during treatment.

2 Where possible a bactericidal drug should be chosen in preference to a bacteristatic drug.

3 Combinations of antibiotics should be avoided except (a) to treat genuine mixed infections, (b) to deter the emergence of drug resistance and (c) in a few cases, e.g. *Strept. viridans* (p. 126), where a certain combination is of proven effectiveness. Any combination should, if at all possible, consist exclusively of bactericidal drugs.

4 A hypersensitivity reaction to an antibiotic will occur with any closely related antibiotic. This *cross-sensitivity* is seen, for example, with all penicillins, and sometimes between the penicillins and cephalosporins.

5 Sloughs and pus must be evacuated surgically; antibiotics alone are inadequate.

6 Antibiotics have great powers both for good and for bad; the good affects the patient, the bad may affect others as well (p. 124). These drugs should therefore never be given without the most careful deliberation.

DRUGS ACTING ON THE NERVOUS SYSTEM

A very large number of drugs are used for their actions on the nervous system. Many are needed in the ICU and staff should know the main characteristics of those used. A complete description of every drug is unnecessary, because they can be classified, according to their actions, into five groups.

1 Hypnotics

An hypnotic drug is one whose main action is to promote sleep. In ordinary doses hypnotics do not relieve pain, and when lack of sleep is due to pain they are of little value. On the other hand, many hypnotics relieve anxiety, and therefore help insomnia which is due to anxiety. Drugs which specifically relieve anxiety without necessarily inducing drowsiness or sleep form a separate group, described later.

Barbiturates

Actions

1 *Depression of the central nervous system.* This may range, according to the dose given, from mild sedation to deep and even fatal coma. Barbiturate-induced sleep is not the same as natural sleep, and withdrawal of these drugs is often followed by a period of readjustment during which insomnia is common.
2 Sometimes *excitation* is seen instead of depression, and the patient behaves as if drunk. This effect depends partly upon the circumstances in which the drug is given; if the patient is already excited, or is prevented from going to sleep, excitation is more likely to occur. A different hypnotic must be chosen.
3 Big doses cause *anaesthesia*, but ordinary doses do not diminish sensitivity to pain. However, thiopentone is a barbiturate which is used only as an intravenous anaesthetic.
4 *Respiratory depression* (p. 87) occurs in proportion to the depth of sleep induced. Mild respiratory depression occurs during even natural sleep and it is doubtful whether barbiturates depress breathing independently of their effect upon consciousness.
5 *The blood pressure and heart rate* fall slightly with ordinary

doses, as they do in natural sleep. With bigger doses, respiratory failure appears before cardiovascular effects become marked. However, in a deeply unconscious patient kept alive by IPPV (p. 250), severe hypotension due to direct depression of the myocardium may be seen.

6 Phenobarbitone and a very few other barbiturates are *anticonvulsants*, in that they suppress the abnormal discharges in the brain which are the basis of epileptic fits.

Preparations

Phenobarbitone is the barbiturate most often used in the ICU. An oral dose (30 to 200 mg) has effects which last for 12 hr or more. Intramuscular injection (up to 200 mg) has a more rapid effect.

Side-effects

1 *Excitation* has been mentioned.
2 *Allergic reactions*, consisting of skin rashes, fever, liver damage and anaemia. Patients with a history of asthma or urticaria are more likely than others to develop allergy to barbiturates.
3 The rather rare disease *porphyria* is aggravated by barbiturates. Its main features are abdominal pain, psychosis, and peripheral neuropathy which may cause respiratory paralysis.

Paraldehyde

Owing to its unpleasant smell and burning taste, paraldehyde is seldom given by mouth. Rectally, 3 to 8 ml in twice this volume of olive oil or saline is well absorbed, taking 30 min to produce maximal sedation. Intramuscular injection may cause necrosis of muscle and the formation of an abscess, and should be avoided. Paraldehyde can be given intravenously in doses of 1 to 4 ml, injected slowly, and by this route it is used to help to control convulsions. It is not clear whether paraldehyde is a specific anticonvulsant or not.

The safety of paraldehyde should not be taken for granted. Large doses produce deep sleep and depression of the respiration and circulation. A special hazard arises in the use of old stocks of the drug, which may contain poisonous impurities due to slow deterioration.

2   Drugs used to relieve anxiety

Benzodiazepines

These are nowadays very widely used in the treatment of anxiety. They include *diazepam* and *lorazepam*. In ordinary doses these drugs relieve anxiety without causing drowsiness. The patient can stay awake if he wishes, but he can go to sleep more easily. In bigger doses these drugs are hypnotic and may produce deep sleep. Respiratory depression is variable, and may be minimal even after big doses. In general, the safety margin is wide.

Diazepam is often used in the ICU to alleviate postoperative anxiety and restlessness. Diazepam does not relieve pain, but in repeated intravenous doses of 5 to 10 mg it is an effective and safe sedative. Given with a narcotic analgesic it may allow a smaller dose of the latter to suffice. Diazepam is also an anticonvulsant.

Nitrazepam, although chemically a member of this group, is primarily an hypnotic.

Phenothiazines

This large group of drugs has numerous actions apart from the relief of anxiety, but is conveniently included here.

Chlorpromazine is the prototype of phenothiazine drugs. It has the following actions:

1   *Sedation*, from which arousal is easy after ordinary doses. Though rousable and rational, however, the patient shows little emotional reaction to events and seems indifferent to stimuli which would normally provoke his response; thus pain is felt but does not have its normal 'significance' to the patient. This is called a *neuroleptic* action.

2   *Spontaneous movement* is reduced. Chlorpromazine is not however an anticonvulsant.

3   Chlorpromazine has an *autonomic blocking action* and also blocks the action of *histamine* (see p. 132).

4   *Baroreceptor reflexes* (p. 56) are weakened.

5   The *myocardium is depressed*, and with actions 3 and 4 this may cause a marked fall in blood pressure.

6   *Vomiting is suppressed* by a central action.

7   The *effects of many other drugs*, including morphine, are enhanced.

Dosage. 25 to 50 mg by intramuscular injection. Subcutaneous injection is painful and intravenous injection often causes hypotension which may be profound in hypovolaemic patients.

Uses. Chlorpromazine is sometimes used for surgical premedication. Its widespread action is rather a disadvantage in other applications.

Promethazine has marked sedative and antihistaminic activity, but its other actions are slight. Its chief use is for sedation, including surgical premedication. The dose is 25 to 50 mg by mouth or intramuscularly.

Prochlorperazine is mainly used to suppress vomiting (5 to 10 mg intramuscularly) or nausea (5 to 25 mg orally). It often causes restlessmess but is almost free from the cardiovascular actions of chlorpromazine.

3   Narcotic-analgesic drugs

Morphine

Actions

1 *Analgesia,* even in doses which do not markedly affect consciousness.
2 *Sedation, sleep or coma,* depending on the dose.
3 *Relief from anxiety,* which produces a sense of well-being and helps to promote addiction.
4 *Respiratory depression,* and a *fall in blood pressure* even in doses which do not cause sleep.
5 *Depression of the cough centre* which favours the retention of bronchial secretions.
6 *Constriction of the pupils.*
7 *Constipation* and *retention of urine* in the bladder.
8 *Vomiting* is common.
   Tolerance to all these actions develops rapidly, and the dose must be increased to produce the same effect.

Contra-indications. Morphine should be used cautiously, or not at all, in patients with asthma, chronic bronchitis and emphysema, and severe obesity. In all of these respiratory depression is dangerous.

The effects of morphine are enhanced by phenothiazines and other drugs.

Dosage. 5 to 20 mg intramuscularly. Smaller, intravenous doses, repeated more frequently, may achieve sedation and analgesia without undue respiratory depression.

Papaveretum

This is a preparation containing morphine with other substances from the opium poppy. Dose for dose it has a slightly less depressant action than morphine and may cause vomiting less readily. Approximately 2 mg of papaveretum has the same effect as 1 mg of morphine.

Pethidine (Meperidine)

This synthetic drug has actions very like those of morphine in equivalent doses (10 mg morphine equals 100 mg pethidine). Pethidine does not markedly constrict the pupils, and does not often cause vomiting. It does not usually lead to constipation and suppresses cough less than morphine does. Its action is also shorter. It has an atropine-like action which results in tachycardia and the relaxation of hollow viscera (p. 32).

Pentazocine

Although chemically related to morphine, pentazocine causes addiction less readily, and respiratory depression and vomiting are less marked than with morphine. Pain is relieved almost as well. Pentazocine actually antagonizes morphine, but not nearly as effectively as nalorphine. The dose is 30 mg intramuscularly.

Nalorphine and naloxone

These drugs are also related to morphine. When given alone nalorphine has analgesic, autonomic and respiratory depressant effects similar to those of morphine and may cause hallucinations. Curiously it is a powerful antagonist of other narcotics when given with them and may thus be used to reverse the effects of an overdose of morphine, papaveretum or pethidine.

Naloxone (0·4 mg IV) is a potent narcotic antagonist which has no narcotic effects when given alone.

4 Anticonvulsants

Generalized convulsions, whether due to the disease we call 'epilepsy' or to definable causes such as cerebral oedema or anoxia, have a common basis in the paroxysmal discharge of abnormal impulses in the brain. These are revealed in the electroencephalogram and can be damped down or suppressed by several drugs, of which diazepam, phenobarbitone, paraldehyde and phenytoin are the most important. The therapeutic use of these drugs in controlling convulsions is discussed on p. 209.

Phenytoin (Diphenylhydantoin)

Unlike phenobarbitone, phenytoin has little sedative action in doses big enough to suppress fits. Instead, it is apt to cause irritability, unsteadiness, tremor and double vision, and when treatment is prolonged it may give rise to swelling of the gums and anaemia. The normal dose is 400 mg daily, but bigger doses may be necessary for short periods. If convulsions 'break through' treatment with phenytoin they are likely to be severe and phenytoin is therefore commonly used in combination with phenobarbitone.

Phenytoin is also effective in suppressing cardiac arrhythmias (p. 111).

5 Local anaesthetics

Several substances, when applied locally to the surface of a nerve, prevent the conduction of impulses along it. Motor nerves are affected as well as sensory nerves; but small nerve fibres, such as the ones carrying pain impulses, are affected more than the large motor fibres and those carrying other sensations. These substances are used in the ICU to induce anaesthesia of small areas for minor surgical procedures and to cause more extensive regional anaesthesia by blockade of one or more large nerves. Intercostal nerve block and epidural anaesthesia are the commonest ICU applications of regional blockade.

Lignocaine (Lidocaine)

This is the most widely used local anaesthetic, acting within a few minutes of injection and lasting up to 3 hours. It is injected as a 0·5 to 2·0 per cent soultion, usually accompanied by adrenaline to counteract the vasodilator action of lignocaine and thus prevent rapid dispersal of the anaesthetic. Up to 500 mg of lignocaine with adrenaline may be given safely to an adult.

Lignocaine is also used intravenously for its powerful suppression of cardiac arrhythmias.

CORTICOSTEROIDS

Several substances are secreted by the cortex of the suprarenal gland. They belong to a chemical group called *steroids* and are therefore termed *corticosteroids*. They may be grouped as follows:
1   *Cortisol* (hydrocortisone), with effects mainly on carbohydrate metabolism and in the protection of the body against stress.
2   *Aldosterone* with effects mainly on sodium reabsorption in the distal tubules of the kidney (p. 93).
3   *Sex hormones*, mainly male (androsterone), but also small amounts of female (oestrogens and progestogens).

Cortisol

The rate of secretion of cortisol, but not of aldosterone, depends on stimulation of the suprarenal by another hormone produced by the pituitary gland. This is adrenocorticotrophic hormone (ACTH), which is secreted in response to need, largely via connections between the pituitary gland and the brain. In addition to this regulation, an increase in circulating cortisol diminishes, and a fall stimulates, the secretion of ACTH. The system is therefore partly self-regulating. Under ordinary conditions 25 to 50 mg of cortisol is secreted daily. In acute stress, such as trauma or severe infection, the secretion of cortisol may exceed 300 mg daily.

The precise way in which cortisol protects against various kinds of stress is not known. The following are its main observable effects:
1   Increase of glycogen stores by conversion of protein to carbohydrate. Protein breakdown is increased. Insulin is antagonized and the blood sugar may increase.

2 The distribution of body fat is altered; this effect includes the rounded 'moon-face' of prolonged cortisol treatment.

3 The actions of adrenaline and noradrenaline (p. 32) are enhanced.

4 The inflammatory response to bacterial, chemical and other stimuli is reduced by cortisol.

5 The immune response to foreign substances (allergy), or to foreign cells, is diminished or suppressed.

6 Owing to protein breakdown, bone loses its framework, calcium is lost, osteoporosis occurs and fractures may result.

7 Cortisol, and most of its therapeutic substitutes, have enough aldosterone-like activity to be a disadvantage in prolonged treatment. Sodium is retained and potassium is lost from the body.

Indications for treatment with corticosteroids

In the ICU, steroids are used in the following circumstances:

1 When adrenocortical secretion is deficient.

a Disease of the suprarenal glands.

b Suppression of the suprarenal glands by previous treatment with steroids.

2 In various conditions of stress.

a Asthma (p. 262).

b Shock (p. 192), especially when due to Gram-negative septicaemia or anaphylaxis.

3 To reduce or prevent tissue swelling.

a In cerebral oedema (p. 209).

b After inhalation of gastric contents (p. 242).

c Following prolonged endotracheal intubation, especially in infants and children.

In groups **2** and **3**, massive doses (1000 mg or more of cortisol or equivalent) may be given. In practice, dexamethasone or methylprednisolone are often preferred to cortisol, since they act more rapidly. They also cause less disturbance of sodium and potassium balance.

Side-effects of steroids

1 *Suprarenal suppression.* ACTH secretion by the pituitary gland is reduced or even abolished by increased amounts of circulating steroids. When these are given, therefore, the suprarenal gland lacks its normal stimulation and rapidly shrinks from disuse. Should treatment suddenly stop, a state of acute suprarenal insufficiency quickly develops. Also, the steroid-treated patient cannot respond to infections or other stress by increasing steroid output from his own suprarenals; the dose of steroid must therefore be increased until the stress subsides.

2 *Infection may be masked* by the anti-inflammatory effect of administered steroid, and the depression of the body's defences may allow infection to spread widely before it is detected.

3 *Fractures*, especially of vertebrae, often occur during prolonged treatment.

4 Serious *depletion of potassium* may occur, with retention of sodium and precipitation of cardiac failure in patients so at risk.

5 *Pitting oedema* without cardiac failure may result from an increase in the permeability of capillaries to water.

Drugs used in steroid treatment include the following.

Drug	Approximate equivalent dosage (mg)
Cortisone	25
Cortisol (hydrocortisone)	20
Prednisolone	5
Prednisone	5
Betamethasone	0·75
Dexamethasone	0·75

Aldosterone

The promotion of Na retention by aldosterone is an effect rarely required therapeutically. In adrenocortical insufficiency however, it may be necessary to add a salt-retaining steroid to the replacement doses of cortisol-like steroid. Aldosterone itself is not used, but *fludrocortisone* is given and acts similarly.

The anatagonism of aldosterone by spironolactone is much more often used therapeutically (p. 108).

Sex hormones of the suprarenal

These do not play any part in intensive care. However, there is a similar group of steroids which has only weak sex effects but strong metabolic effects, promoting the building of body protein. These are the so-called *anabolic steroids* of which *norethandrolone* is an example, and they are sometimes used to promote nutrition after surgical operations.

3   Clinical Aspects of Intensive Care

8 Cardiac Arrhythmias

The term *arrhythmia* literally means 'absence of rhythm', but it is used to indicate any abnormality of rate, regularity, origin of impulse or conduction. Recognition and treatment of arrhythmias are discussed in this chapter. Anti-arrhythmic drugs have already been described (p. 111).

The electrocardiogram

With each heartbeat, the excitation wave (p. 41) sets up small electrical voltages which can be detected at any part of the body. The electrocardiogram is a record of changes in voltage at a particular site compared with a chosen reference site or combination of sites. Essentially, therefore, two electrodes are required, to record

The standard set of leads comprises:

	Electrode 1	Electrode 2
Standard limb leads		
Lead 1	Left arm (LA)	Right arm (RA)
Lead 2	Left leg (LL)	RA
Lead 3	LL	LA
'Augmented unipolar' limb leads		
Lead AVR	RA	Connected LA and LL
Lead AVL	LA	Connected RA and LL
Lead AVF	LL	Connected RA and LA
Precordial leads		
Leads V3R to V6	See Fig. 21	Connected RA, LA and LL
Miscellaneous leads		

Leads V6R to V4R are sometimes used when the heart is displaced to the right. Other chest leads, oesophageal and intracardiac leads are sometimes used for special purposes.

141

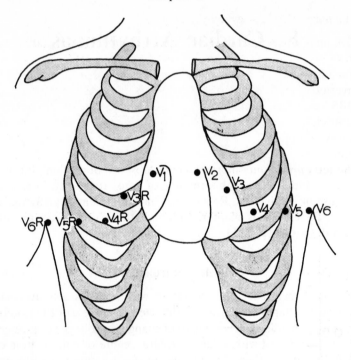

Fig. 21 ECG electrode positions.
V_1 4th intercostal space to the right of the sternum
V_2 4th intercostal space to the left of the sternum
V_3 midway between V_2 and V_4
V_4 5th intercostal space mid-clavicular line
V_5 anterior axillary line at the same level as V_4
V_6 mid-axillary line at the same level as V_4
V_7 posterior axillary line at the same level as V_4
V_3R to V_6R similar to V_3 to V_6, but over the right chest

an ECG. A third electrode, usually attached to the right leg, is connected to earth.

The site of the recording electrodes determines the kind of record obtained, and certain electrode positions have become standard. The normal patterns expected from the electrode combinations or 'leads' have been very thoroughly established.

The normal electrocardiogram (Fig. 22)

Five main deflections ('waves') accompany each heartbeat. The P wave occurs as the excitation wave (the wave of depolarisation) spreads through the atria and is often best seen in lead 2. It is inverted in lead AVR but is usually upright in the other leads. The QRS 'complex' occurs as the excitation wave spreads through the ventricles. The Q wave is small and inverted, and may be absent; the R wave is upright and the S wave is inverted. The T wave is upright in most leads; it represents the recovery of the ventricles from the passage of the excitation wave.

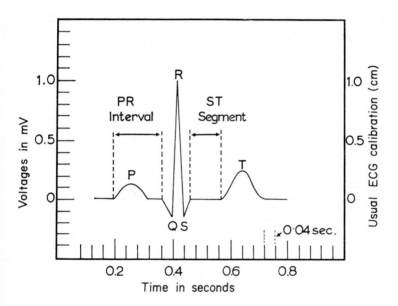

Fig. 22 Normal ECG deflections (diagrammatic).

The appearance of the QRS complex varies to some extent from lead to lead and from patient to patient but normal patterns are readily recognizable and a typical example is shown in Fig. 23. Note that over the right ventricle (leads V3R and V1) the QRS deflection is predominantly negative (below the line) while over the left ventricle (leads V5 and V6) the deflection is predominantly positive (above the line).

The interval from the beginning of the P wave to the beginning of the QRS (the PR interval) is a measure of the time taken for the excitation wave to pass through the atria, the AV node, the bundle of His and the right and left bundles, and is normally 0·2 sec or less. The duration of the QRS complex is normally 0·12 sec or less, and it is a measure of the time taken for the excitation wave to spread through the ventricles.

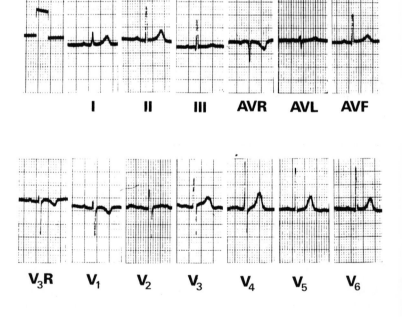

Fig. 23 Normal ECG.

ECG paper is marked in mm with a thick line every 5 mm. It is usually driven at a rate of 25 mm per sec. Each mm represents, therefore, 0·04 sec and 5 mm represents 0·2 sec. The arbitrary limits of the normal resting heart rate are 60 and 100 beats per minute; less than 60 is termed *bradycardia* and more than 100 *tachycardia*. The rate is quickly measured from the ECG by counting the number of QRS complexes in 6 sec (15 cm) and multiplying by 10. Alternatively one can divide the number of thick lines between successive R waves into 300; for example in Fig. 25 the rate is about 300/2·5 = 120. In practice most people prefer to use a rate-ruler for quick assessment.

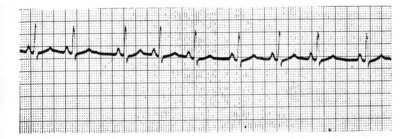

Fig. 24 Sinus arrhythmia. Note the slight variation in the distance between successive R waves.

The term *'sinus rhythm'* is used to indicate that the cardiac impulse starts in the sinus node and spreads without interruption to the ventricles. If the heart rate is carefully measured from beat to beat it is rarely found to be absolutely regular. Sometimes the rate increases with each inspiration and decreases with each expiration; this is called *sinus arrhythmia* (Fig. 24). It is very common in young people and is not abnormal.

Wandering pacemaker is occasionally seen (Fig. 25). The pacemaker apparently shifts from one site to another producing abrupt changes in the P wave and the PR interval. This rhythm is not strictly normal but does not call for treatment. It often arises when the sinus node is depressed, for example with the stress of cardiac surgery and subsequent abnormalities in blood gases and electro-

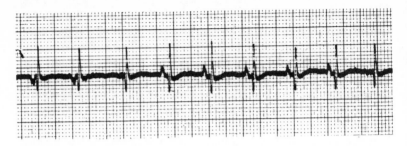

Fig. 25 Wandering pacemaker. Note the abrupt changes in the form of the P waves.

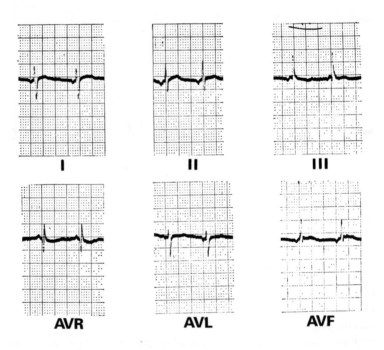

Fig. 26 Junctional rhythm. Because the electrical impulse spreads in an abnormal fashion from the region of the AV node to the atria, P waves are abnormal, being inverted in leads 1, 2, 3 and AVF and upright in AVR. The QRS complexes are normal. The rate is 100 per min, but higher rates are common.

lytes. Many of the impulses are likely to be of junctional origin. Under these circumstances the *junctional pacemaker* may take over directly (Fig. 26). The term *nodal* was formerly used to describe beats originating in the region of the A-V node. It was subsequently demonstrated that these arise in conducting tissue on either side of the node, rather than in the node itself. The term *junctional* is therefore preferred, indicating an origin from conduction tissue at the junction of atrial and ventricular myocardium.

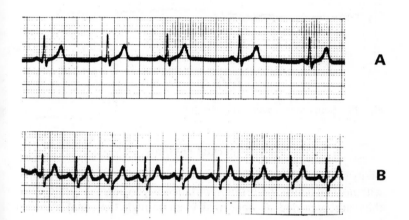

Fig. 27 Sinus tachycardia: (A), tracing at rest, rate about 60 per min. (B), after exercise, rate about 105 per min. P waves and QRS complexes are similar to those recorded at rest.

Sinus tachycardia (Fig. 27) denotes sinus rhythm with a resting rate greater than 100 per min. It is a normal accompaniment of exercise, pain, fright or anxiety, and is part of the response to a low cardiac output (p. 190). It also occurs in fever, hyperthyroidism and with the administration of isoprenaline or adrenaline. It is not an abnormal rhythm.

Sinus bradycardia (Fig. 28), with the resting rate less than 60 per min, is often seen in fit athletes. It may be due to excessive vagal stimulation as in fainting, alimentary distension or after myocardial infarction. Bradycardia due to vagal stimulation may be extreme and the heart may even stop; it may contribute importantly to a low cardiac output and is abolished by atropine. Sinus bradycardia also occurs in hypothyroidism and sometimes in digitalis poisoning. In the ICU the most common cause is the preoperative administration of beta-receptor blocking drugs.

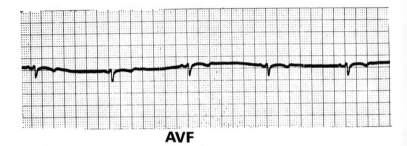

AVF

Fig. 28   Sinus bradycardia, rate 44 per min.

Abnormal rhythms

Many of the rhythms described below occur at some time in people with normal hearts, reverting spontaneously to normal. Despite this they are regarded as abnormal even though they may cause a healthy person no inconvenience.

An *ectopic beat* is one which originates at a site other than the sinus node. It may arise at a supraventricular or ventricular site. Usually the abnormal beat is *premature,* in that it comes before the next normal sinus beat would be expected. In *supraventricular ectopic beats,* the QRS complex looks the same as it does in sinus beats but the P wave is abnormal or concealed in the QRS complex. In *ventricular* ectopic beats, since the excitation wave follows an abnormal pathway in the ventricle, the QRS complex looks abnormal. Ectopic beats arising from more than one focus may be seen and are described as 'multifocal' ectopic beats.

Ectopic beats, whether supraventricular or ventricular, may arise in one of two ways:
1   One region of the heart may be hyperexcitable, and discharge prematurely; spread of the excitation wave from this *abnormal focus* produces the ectopic beat.

2 A *re-entrant* circuit may occur. An example, in the region of the A-V node, is shown in Fig. 29. Over part of its course the conduction pathway divides into two alternative routes. The depolarization wave passes down to the ventricle through one route (labelled 1, Fig. 29) but, as it passes the distal junction of the divided pathway, it sends a simultaneous wave of depolarization back up the second route (2) to the atrium. An atrial ectopic beat is therefore produced.

Atrium

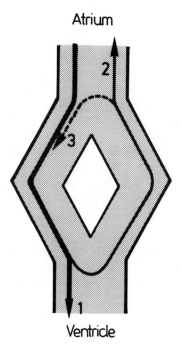

Ventricle

Fig. 29 Basis for re-entrant arrhythmias in the region of the A-V node (see text). A continuous cycle develops around the pathway. Usually a retrograde atrial impulse (end of pathway 2) and a ventricular impulse (end of pathway 1) occur with each cycle. If, say, alternate impulses to the ventricle are blocked, a supraventricular tachycardia with 2:1 block is seen in the ECG.

When the proximal junction is reached by wave (2) the first route may be able to conduct again. If so, a further wave of depolarization will pass once more down to the ventricle (3). A continuous cycle can therefore be set up and the result is a supraventricular tachycardia. Usually an atrial and ventricular complex are seen with each cycle. Sometimes there is an intermittent block in one limb so that, for example, the ventricular complex may be seen only with each second cycle; in the ECG this then appears as a supraventricular arrhythmia with 2 : 1 block.

The same type of mechanism occurs in the Wolff-Parkinson-White syndrome but here the impulse often travels down the normal pathway and returns through an abnormal pathway which may be many centimetres from the A-V node. Small re-entrant pathways also occur in the ventricles, producing ventricular ectopic beats and ventricular tachycardia.

Ectopic beats may occur in the absence of demonstrable heart disease, especially after heavy consumption of tobacco or coffee. Ventricular ectopic beats are more likely than supraventricular beats to denote cardiac disease, and are therefore more important. The patient may be unaware that an ectopic beat has occurred, but sometimes he feels that his heart misses a beat and then gives a powerful thump, so that his 'heart turns over'; this kind of palpitation is familiar to most normal people. When a premature beat occurs, the ventricle has less time to fill and therefore ejects less

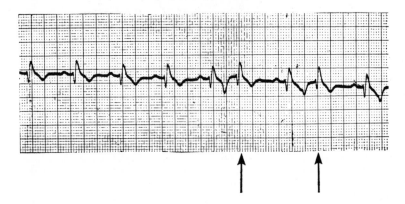

Fig. 30 Supraventricular ectopic beats. The QRS complexes of the ectopic beats (arrowed) are identical with those of the sinus beats and follow premature, inverted P waves which distort the preceding T wave. These are junctional ectopic beats. (This record also shows right bundle-branch block.)

blood. At the pulse, the beat comes early and feels weak. A very early beat cannot be felt at all, and a beat is 'missed'. These events can also be seen in the arterial pressure tracing. Infrequent ectopic beats are harmless and rarely merit treatment. When heart disease is present, however, frequent ectopic beats may herald the onset of supraventricular or ventricular tachycardias.

Following the above general account, arrhythmias are best considered in relation to their origin.

Supraventricular arrhythmias

Supraventricular ectopic beats (Fig. 30). Regular sinus rhythm is interrupted by premature beats. Because the excitation wave starts at an abnormal site and spreads through the atria in an abnormal fashion, the P waves in the ECG have a different form from those seen with sinus beats. For the same reason the PR interval is

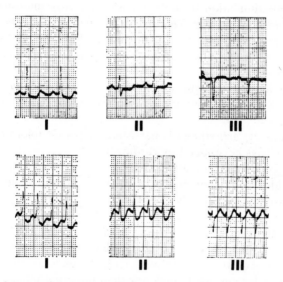

Fig. 31 Supraventricular tachycardia. Upper trace, sinus rhythm, rate 83 per min. Lower trace, supraventricular tachycardia, rate 200 per min. P waves are abnormal but the QRS complexes are the same as those seen in sinus rhythm. The ST segments are depressed during the rapid cardiac action.

abnormal; this is particularly so with junctional ectopic beats when the P wave may be concealed in the QRS or follow it. However, the QRS complex is unchanged unless, as sometimes happens, bundle branch block occurs with the ectopic beat.

Supraventricular tachycardia (usually re-entrant) has a rate of about 160 to 250 beats per min (Fig. 31). Usually there is an atrial and a ventricular complex to each cycle but sometimes, especially when the tachycardia is induced by digitalis, some ventricular responses are blocked and each second, third or fourth beat is conducted. The QRS complex is normal unless a separate abnormality, for example bundle branch block, is present.

Supraventricular tachycardia usually starts and stops abruptly. The term *paroxysmal tachycardia* is sometimes used but the adjective 'paroxysmal' adds little to understanding or description. It is not serious if the heart can tolerate the high rate. It may affect otherwise normal hearts.

Treatment
1 Vagal stimulation by reflex action may stop the attack. The patient may learn the Valsalva or Müller manoeuvre (strong expiratory or inspiratory effort against a closed airway) or exert pressure on the eyeballs or on the carotid sinus just behind the angle of the jaw.
2 Should these measures fail, verapamil will usually stop the attack. Digoxin, disopyramide or phenytoin are also effective in many cases.
3 Where the arrhythmia is persistent or poorly tolerated it can almost always be stopped by cardioversion.
4 To prevent further attacks in a patient prone to them, disopyramide or quinidine may be given indefinitely. The newer drug amiodarone is particularly effective in prevention.

Atrial flutter (Fig. 32). Here the atrial rate is usually 250 to 350 per min and in some ECG leads, especially lead 2, P waves have a 'saw-tooth' appearance. Atrioventricular block is common so that the ventricular rate is often slower than the atrial rate.

Atrial flutter may affect otherwise normal hearts but more often it is caused by the same conditions which produce atrial fibrillation. *Treatment and prevention* are the same as for supraventricular tachycardia but cardioversion is required more frequently.

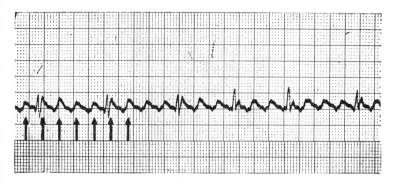

Fig. 32 Atrial flutter. The atrial rate is 270 per min and the P waves (arrowed) have a saw-toothed configuration. The ventricles respond to every 3rd or 4th atrial complex giving a ventricular rate of about 85 per min.

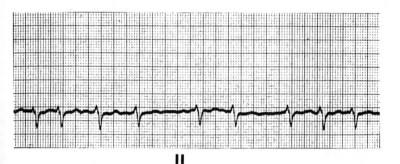

Fig. 33 Atrial fibrillation. Atrial complexes are irregular and the rate is high. The ventricles respond erratically giving an irregular ventricular rhythm with a rate of about 85 per min.

Atrial fibrillation (Fig. 33). In this condition the atrial contraction is ineffective and totally uncoordinated. Irregular small atrial waves are seen in the ECG at rates of 350 to 700 per min. The ventricles cannot respond at this rate, and beat quite irregularly at up to 200 per min. Occasionally this arrhythmia affects otherwise normal hearts, but usually it complicates longstanding coronary artery disease, rheumatic heart disease (especially mitral stenosis) or thyrotoxicosis. The patient notices irregular palpitations; the pulse is totally irregular and, when rapid, its rate is less than the heart rate. This difference, between the heart rate counted by auscultation or on the ECG and the pulse rate felt at the wrist, is called the *pulse deficit.*

Complication. Clot tends to form in the atria, and pulmonary and systemic emboli are common.

Treatment
1 In most cases sinus rhythm may be restored by cardioversion If the arrhythmia has been present for two weeks or more, anti-coagulants are introduced before taking this step. Treatment is then usually started with disopyramide or quinidine before cardioversion and sometimes sinus rhythm is restored by one of these drugs alone. After reversion the drug is continued indefinitely in an attempt to keep the patient in sinus rhythm. In long standing atrial fibrillation, or with severe cardiac disease, sinus rhythm can seldom be maintained for long.
2 The atrial fibrillation may have to be accepted, and its risks minimized by (a) digitalization to control the ventricular rate and cardiac failure, and (b) anticoagulant treatment to reduce the risks of embolism.

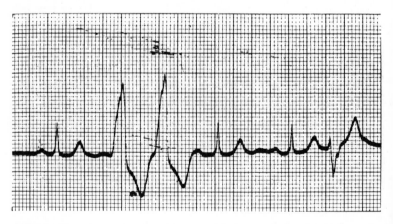

Fig. 34 Ventricular ectopic beats. Two forms of QRS are seen in the ectopic beats which are therefore of multifocal origin.

Ventricular arrhythmias

Ventricular ectopic beats (ventricular extrasystoles) (Fig. 34). Although ventricular ectopic beats may occur in otherwise normal hearts, they occur more frequently in the presence of significant myocardial disease. The ventricular origin of the ectopic beats is shown by the fact that they are not preceded by a P wave and the QRS contour is abnormal. In the ICU they occur especially in two situations:

1 When cardiac output is low after operation, especially when potassium depletion is present and the patient is digitalized.

2 After myocardial infarction, when even a small infarct may give rise to an irritable focus which assumes the role of pacemaker for one or more beats at a time. One of the functions of monitoring in coronary care units is to detect and deal with ventricular ectopic beats judged to be of a threatening nature.

Treatment

1 Ventricular ectopic beats can often be reduced in frequency with procainamide, mexilitine, disopyramide or quinidine.

2 More vigorous therapy is required.

a If ectopic beats occur in runs, often called salvos (Fig. 35).

b If they occur on the T wave of the previous complex (Fig. 36).

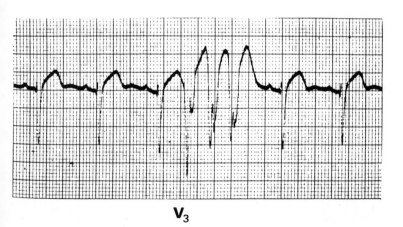

V₃

Fig. 35 Ventricular ectopic beats. A salvo of 3 ectopic beats is seen.

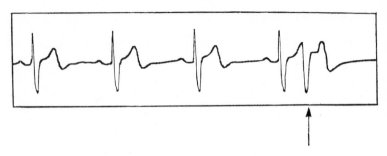

Fig. 36 Ventricular ectopic beats, R on T. The ectopic beat (arrow) falls on the T wave of the previous sinus beat.

In each of these situations the ectopic beats are more liable to lead to ventricular fibrillation or tachycardia. In most cases intravenous infusion of lignocaine will suppress the ectopic beats. If this is ineffective procainamide, bretyllium or mexiletine may be added. Intravenous amiodarone is used increasingly in resistant cases.

If the ectopic beats are thought to be due to digitalis this drug must be stopped. While digitalis may cause irregular ectopic beats, the presence of coupled beats, in which sinus and ectopic beats alternate (also called bigeminy), is particularly suggestive of digitalis toxicity (Fig. 37). In addition to withholding digitalis, treatment with lignocaine, phenytoin or propranolol may be needed. Administration of potassium chloride if often necessary.

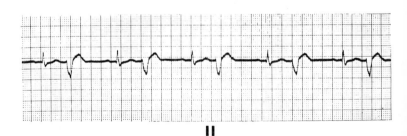

II

Fig. 37 Coupled ventricular ectopic beats. Sinus and ectopic beats alternate.

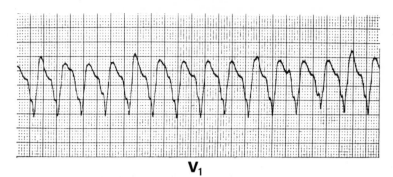

V₁

Fig. 38 Ventricular tachycardia. The rhythm is fairly regular but the QRS complexes are abnormal and P waves cannot be identified.

Ventricular tachycardia (Fig. 38). The ectopic ventricular focus assumes total control of the rhythm. P waves are usually absent or at least difficult to identify, the QRS complex is wide and distorted and the rhythm is relatively regular. The rate is usually between 150 and 250 per min although lower rates may be seen, particularly after myocardial infarction. When the rate is high the cardiac output and arterial pressure often fall sharply.

Complicatiions

(1) Rapid progress of cardiac failure, and (2) development of ventricular fibrillation.

Treatment

1 Rapid ventricular tachycardia is an emergency requiring urgent treatment. DC cardioversion (p. 115) is usually required. If the patient develops hypotension and begins to lose consciousness this procedure must be carried out immediately.
2 If the arrhythmia is well tolerated and does not produce hypotension there is usually time to attempt reversion with a lignocaine infusion (p. 112). The slow 'accelerated idioventricular rhythm', seen after myocardial infarction, may not require active treatment (p. 232).

3 If severe hypotension has occurred, lactic acidosis is likely to have developed and sodium bicarbonate, 1 to 3 mmol per kg body weight, should be injected intravenously.
4 Digitalis must usually be stopped.
5 Potassium depletion must be countered appropriately.
6 After successful restoration of sinus rhythm, the ectopic focus is suppressed with an intravenous infusion of lignocaine, supplemented if necessary with procainamide, mexilitine, disopyramide or propranolol. Subsequently it may be necessary to continue prophylaxis with the oral medication.

It may be difficult to distinguish ventricular tachycardia from supraventricular tachycardia with bundle branch block because the QRS is widened and distorted in the latter condition. Fortunately it is, in general, better tolerated and some clue to the diagnosis may arise with time. Where doubt remains, however, the arrhythmia must usually be regarded as ventricular tachycardia.

Ventricular fibrillation (Fig. 39). When this occurs, circulation stops and the patient loses consciousness; it is a form of 'cardiac arrest' (p. 200). The ECG shows bizarre, irregular and variable QRS complexes and P waves are not seen.

Treatment: See 'Cardiac arrest', p. 201.

Ventricular standstill (ventricular asystole) (Fig. 40). This is the other, less treatable, form of cardiac arrest. It may occur during ventricular fibrillation, or directly after a myocardial infarct, in

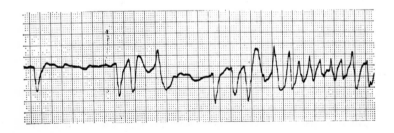

Fig. 39 Ventricular fibrillation. QRS complexes are irregular and bizarre.

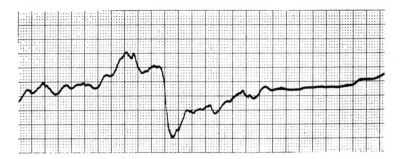

Fig. 40   Ventricular standstill. Ventricular activity ceases. This tracing was recorded 10 seconds after that in Fig. 39.

severe hypotension or in complete heart block. QRS complexes are absent or very infrequent.

Treatment: See 'cardiac arrest', p. 201.

Disorders of conduction

The normal conduction pathway and the production of the normal ECG have been described (p. 41 and p. 143). Although any part of the conduction system can act as a pacemaker, the sinus node normally does so because its 'firing' rate is highest. Thus, for example, junctional tissue normally has no chance to act as pacemaker since it is constantly suppressed by the activation wave from the faster sinus node. If, however, the sinus node is suppressed the junctional tissue may temporarily have the faster firing-rate. Usually this results in a junctional rhythm, the excitation wave spreading both to atria and ventricles. Occasionally the wave does not pass into the atria; the ventricles are then stimulated by the faster junctional pacemaker while the atria are activated by the slower sinus node. This is called *atrioventricular dissociation* and an example is shown in Fig. 41. This arrhythmia which is not uncommon after cardiac surgery, especially in infants, generally reverts to sinus rhythm without treatment.

An entirely different problem arises when damage to the conducting tissue prevents the passage of the normal activation wave from the sinus node. This interference with normal conduction is

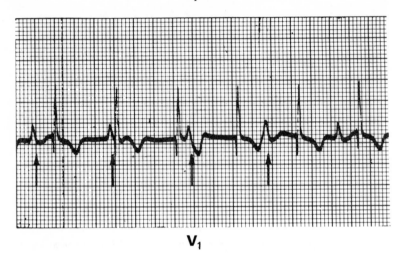

V₁

Fig. 41 A-V dissociation. The atrial rate is 75 (first 4 P waves arrowed) and the ventricular rate is 95 per min. Ventricles and atria therefore contract independently, i.e. they are dissociated.

called 'block'. Damage to the right or left bundle makes the electrical impulse take a roundabout route and so alters the ECG. Damage to both bundle branches, or to the A–V bundle itself, blocks the impulse altogether and produces atrioventricular block.

Bundle branch block

Right bundle branch block (RBBB, Fig. 42). Damage to the right bundle delays the arrival of the excitation wave to the right ventricle. The QRS complex is wider than 0·12 sec. Tall, wide R waves are seen over the right side of the heart (V3R and V1) RBBB is seen in many cardiac disorders, especially with severe right ventricular hypertrophy and in atrial septal defect. During surgical closure of a ventricular septal defect, a stitch may damage the right bundle. An anterior myocardial infarct may do the same.

Treatment. RBBB is in itself harmless, which is fortunate because it cannot be influenced by treatment. Occurring after myocardial

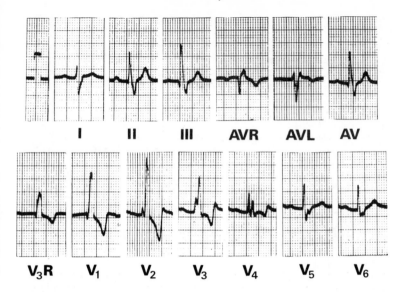

I   II   III   AVR   AVL   AV

V₃R   V₁   V₂   V₃   V₄   V₅   V₆

Fig. 42   Right bundle branch block.

infarction it may progress to complete A–V block (p. 164) and artificial pacing may thus become necessary.

Left bundle branch block (LBBB, Fig. 43). Damage to the left bundle delays the arrival of the excitation wave to the left ventricle. The QRS complex is wider than 0·12 sec. Tall, broad R waves are seen over the left ventricle (V5 and V6). LBBB is commonest in ischaemic heart disease but is often seen in other cardiac conditions.

Treatment: No treatment is possible or necessary.

Atrioventricular block (A–V block)

A–V block may result from damage to the bundle of His or from simultaneous damage to the right and left bundle branches. It may occur as a congenital lesion or as a result of inflammation, infarction or surgical trauma, or from poisoning with drugs, e.g. digitalis. The degree of block varies, and three grades may be recognized:

1   *First degree block* (Fig. 44) is merely delay in A–V conduction.

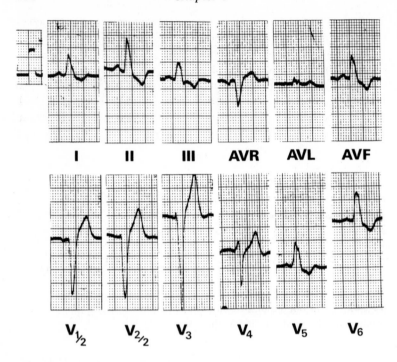

Fig. 43 Left bundle branch block.

The PR interval exceeds 0·2 sec. Specific treatment is seldom necessary but an underlying cause should be sought and dealt with if present (e.g. by stopping digitalis).

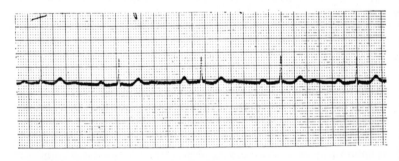

Fig. 44 First degree A-V block. The PR interval is 0·3 sec.

2 *Second degree block.* Here some atrial complexes are not conducted to the ventricles at all, and therefore some P waves are not followed by a QRS complex. Sometimes the PR interval is seen to increase with successive beats until a QRS complex is dropped, then the PR interval abruptly shortens and the cycle is repeated. This is called the *Wenckebach phenomenon* (Fig. 45). It is also called *Mobitz type 1 block.* The block is often quite high in the conduction pathway.

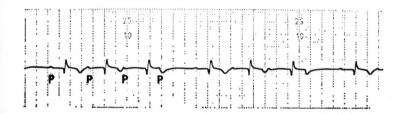

Fig. 45 Second degree A-V block, the Wenckebach phenomenon. The PR interval increases progressively and every 4th atrial impulse is not conducted. This is also called Mobitz type 1 block.

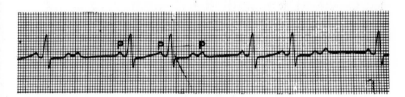

Fig. 46 Second degree A-V block. Mobitz type 2.

Sometimes a QRS complex is dropped abruptly without prior shortening of the PR interval. This is *Mobitz type 2 block* (Fig. 46). Here the block tends to be lower in the conduction tissue and the risk of developing complete heart block is higher than with Mobitz type 1 block.

Withdrawal of digitalis may be needed and treatment with isoprenaline may be indicated. For Mobitz type 2 block a pacemaker must be considered.

3 *Third degree block — 'complete A–V block'* (Fig. 47). All atrial beats are blocked, and a lower pacemaker (in the A–V node or ventricle) takes over the ventricular rhythm. The ventricles beat regularly at a lower rate than the atria and ventricular rates of 30 to 50 are common. In congenital A–V block the rate tends to be more nearly normal. At ventricular rates below 40, cardiac output may be impaired at rest. On exercise, output is even less adequate and syncope results.

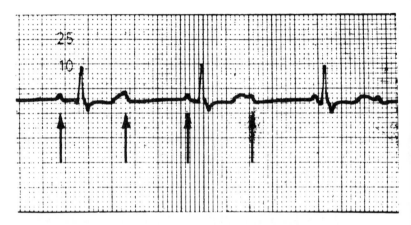

Fig. 47 Complete A-V block. P waves (the first 4 are arrowed) show no relationship to QRS complexes. Atrial rate 108, ventricular rate 52 per min.

Especially at the onset of complete block, the ventricular pacemaker may fail to 'fire' leading to ventricular standstill, sometimes followed by ventricular fibrillation. The patient loses consciousness. This is a *Stokes-Adams attack.* The ventricular pacemaker may recover spontaneously after a short period of asystole; nevertheless Stokes-Adams attacks demand urgent treatment since they are often fatal.

Treatment. Intravenous infusion of isoprenaline (p. 117) may improve conduction when A–V block is intermittent. If the cause is transitory the circulation may thus be maintained until the A–V block disappears. Even if sinus rhythm is not restored isoprenaline may increase the ventricular rate enough to prevent syncopal attacks until either the block disappears or an artificial pacemaker is provided.

When block is prolonged or syncopal attacks are frequent, the heart may have to be 'paced' electrically. A brief, undirectional impulse is applied to an electrode in contact with the heart; this causes an excitation wave to spread from the electrode site to the rest of the myocardium. It is convenient to consider the topic of pacemakers at this point.

Cardiac pacemakers

Indications for pacing

1 Heart block — either complete heart block with a slow rate or intermittent heart block with syncopal turns.
2 An unreliable sinus rhythm. In the sick sinus syndrome bouts of tachycardia (requiring suppressive treatment) alternate with marked sinus bradycardia and periods of sinus arrest. After operation marked sinus bradycardia may be present in patients treated preoperatively with beta blockers and very slow atrial fibrillation may occur particularly in patients with severe mitral valve disease.
3 Postoperatively pacing may be required, even without these indications, in patients with a critically low cardiac output when maintenance of an optimal pulse rate may be essential for survival. As this situation may be difficult to predict, pacing wires are inserted routinely in many patients.

Electrodes

For emergency pacing outside the operating theatre and for long-term pacing, an electrode catheter is normally passed pervenously and lodged in the right ventricle. For both temporary and permanent pacing at operation, electrode wires are normally sewn on to the surface of the heart.

With *pervenous pacing* the catheter may be bipolar, with one electrode at the tip and the other a short distance behind it; the pacing current passes from one electrode through a short segment of myocardium to the other electrode, returning to the pacemaker

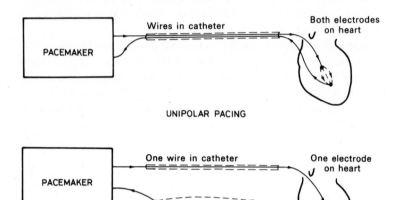

Fig. 48　Diagram to illustrate bipolar and unipolar pacing.

to complete the circuit (Fig. 48). Or it may be *unipolar,* with one electrode at the tip; in this case the current passes from the electrode through the myocardium and body tissues to another electrode sewn under the skin and returns from these to the pacemaker to complete the circuit. The best results are obtained with the negative electrode in contact with the heart. The case of an implanted pacemaker may act as the return electrode. *Epicardial electrodes,* sewn on the surface of the myocardium, are usually unipolar and require a separate return wire.

Temporary pacing

With a pervenous electrode, the ends of the catheter are simply connected with the pacemaker unit. Postoperatively, however, epicardial electrodes are usually employed. There are usually two wires attached to the heart — an atrial electrode and a ventricular electrode. A third wire is sewn into muscle and acts as the return electrode. Three forms of pacing are then possible, depending on requirements.

1 Atrial pacing can be used provided the patient does not have atrial fibrillation or A–V block, to maintain an optimal rate. An added bonus with the atrial wire is that it can be joined to the V lead of an ECG machine, often allowing accurate diagnosis of arrhythmias in difficult cases. (Some surgeons actually insert two atrial wires to allow for a better ECG recording).

2 A–V sequential pacing can be employed where A–V block is present. The atrial stimulus comes 0·1 to 0·15 sec before the ventricular stimulus to maintain the normal sequence of contraction and allow the atrium to prime the ventricle for optimal filling.

3 Where atrial pacing is not practical, an optimal rate can be obtained by ventricular pacing.

Because an external pacemaker unit is employed, the rate can be set at any desired level. The output of the pacemaker (whether measured in voltage or amperage) can be increased to a level to ensure satisfactory pacing. Sometimes a demand mode unit is used, ensuring satisfactory function while the patient is not being directly observed.

Permanent pacing

For most patients pervenous pacing is favoured. A thoracotomy is not required and satisfactory long-term pacing is achieved more frequently. In small children, however, no provision can be made for growth and epicardial pacing may be necessary. Usually this is achieved at thoracotomy but some surgeons use a system of special screw electrodes which can be inserted through a very small incision. The electrode wires can then be curled around to allow for growth. With either the epicardial or pervenous system, the wires are then tracked subcutaneously to be attached to the pacemaker situated in a satisfactory site.

Types of pacing

1 *Fixed-rate pacing.* Here the pacemaker unit continues to produce a regular pacing spike, even if the patient returns to sinus rhythm. Because the rate can be altered in some such units the term *asynchronous* is sometimes preferred, indicating that the patient's own impulse has no effect on the pacemaker.

2 *Demand pacing* (the word *synchronous* pacing is preferred by some). Here a run-down circuit is included and this fires after a predetermined RR interval (i.e. the time between two consecutive R waves); the circuit is reset by any QRS from the patient and therefore the pacing spike is generated only when the patient's rate falls below a given level. This is clearly preferable when the patient might return to sinus rhythm or where his own ventricular rate is sometimes fast. For this reason demand units are usually preferred to fixed-rate units. On the other hand they do have the disadvantage that the run-down circuit will sometimes sense muscular or other interference and so become inhibited when it should be pacing. If this occurs a fixed-rate mode is required.

3   *A–V sequential pacing.* It would obviously be preferable in all patients to have an atrial contraction preceding the ventricular contraction and this is achieved by this type of unit. The disadvantage is that the pacemaker is more complex and failure of part of its function is more likely. It is more difficult to maintain satisfactory atrial pacing than ventricular pacing; if atrial pacing fails the unit reverts to the ventricular mode. Most groups reserve A–V sequential pacing for patients with a particularly low cardiac output where atrial priming of the ventricle is essential.

4   *P-synchronous pacemakers.* In theory this is a still better system, allowing the patient to set his own sinus rate, and timing the ventricular pacing impulse at an appropriate interval after the P wave. This has not yet been shown sufficiently reliable to achieve widespread usage.

5   Special units for the treatment of intractable arrhythmias. Units have been devised which can scan the patient's rhythm and, if a tachycardia develops, produce a critically timed pacing impulse to interrupt the arrhythmia. These are applicable in patients with supraventricular or ventricular arrhythmias but only where detailed electrophysiological study has defined the appropriate timing of the cardioverting or *blocking* impulse. Some pacemaking units, having detected an arrhythmia, pace at a fast rate to achieve fast *overdrive pacing*. A pacemaker discharging at about 150 per min may break into the arrhythmia and capture the rhythm (even though the arrhythmia was faster); sinus rhythm will be restored when the pacemaker switches off. In yet other pacemaker units, a timed impulse can be triggered by a *radio frequency unit*. The patient, feeling an arrhythmia beginning, holds the radio frequency device over the pacemaker to trigger the blocking pulse. These

special units have limited application in some hospitals with special electrophysiological interests and skills. In other hospitals patients with intractable arrhythmias, unresponsive to medication, are considered for surgical treatment.

Programmable units

For all types of units described above, increasingly sophisticated methods of programming have been developed. Programmable pacemakers are so built that some aspect of their function can be altered by a programming unit held close to the pacemaker. The required variable is dialled (for example a given heart rate) and the programming unit emits a train of coded magnetic impulses which reset the pacemaker. The coding is deliberately made relatively complicated so that there is no risk that the pacemaker can be altered by random electro-magnetic fields. Rates can commonly be varied between 50 and 120; output can be varied by increasing the duration of the impulse (the average is around 0·5 msec) or its energy level. Some units may be changed, for example, from A–V sequential to fixed rate pacing. Each level of complexity introduces its own electronic problems and some compromise is required between versatility, reliability and cost. In practice many types of pacemaker units are now available and an attempt is made to find the most suitable unit for each individual patient.

Problems in pacing (Fig. 49)

Failed pacing. In the ICU the likeliest cause for failure to pace is a poor connection in the temporary pacing system. Dislodgement of the wire from the myocardium is less likely.

If, as is now unusual, the patient was being paced pervenously with a bipolar catheter, pacing can sometimes be restored by converting it to a unipolar system, since one of the electrodes often retains good contact with the heart even though the other is unsatisfactory. In an emergency, an ordinary ECG limb lead can be used as the return electrode by leaving one or other of the pacing leads connected to the pacemaker and joining the ECG lead to the other pacemaker terminal, ensuring that good contact with the limb is maintained with electrode paste.

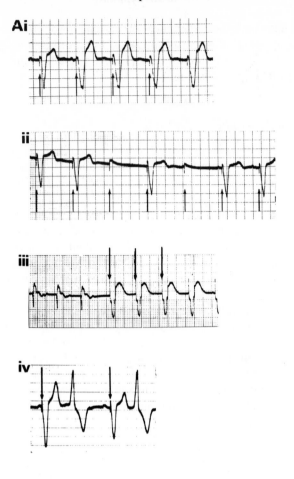

Fig. 49 (*also facing page*) ECGs during cardiac pacing. (A) Ventricular pacing. (i) Fixed rate pacing. Each pacemaker artefact (arrowed in this and subsequent tracings) triggers a QRS complex. (ii) Intermittent pacing failure. The third and fifth pacemaker artefacts fail to capture and are therefore not followed by a QRS complex. (iii) Demand ventricular pacing. The first three complexes are spontaneous idioventricular beats but as soon as there is a pause (in this case only 0·6 seconds) the pacemaker takes over. Usually a longer pause is allowed, but in this patient a fast rate was desired. (iv) Demand ventricular pacing interrupted by ventricular premature beats. The demand unit is set to pace with an R-R interval of 0·9 seconds, but the unit senses the QRS complex for the ectopic beat, discharging again 0·9 seconds after it.

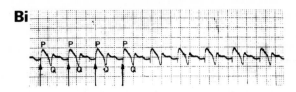

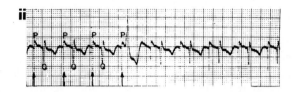

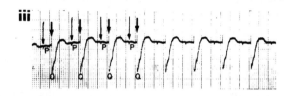

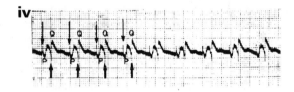

(B) Atrial and A-V sequential pacing. (i) Typical appearance of atrial pacing. Atrial pacemaker artefacts are arrowed. P = P wave. Q = QRS complex. (ii) Another example of atrial pacing. The P and QRS complexes vary according to the lead selected. One ectopic ventricular complex replaces one conducted ventricular complex. (iii) A-V sequential pacing. The atrial and ventricular pacing artefacts are both inconspicuous and a different lead selection might be necessary to show them clearly. (iv) A-V sequential pacing. The atrial and ventricular pacing artefacts are more easily seen in this patient.

With the standard epicardial system pacing may be restored by increasing the output of the pacemaker. If this is unsuccessful further steps for emergency pacing may be required but fortunately this is a rare event.

Frequent ventricular ectopic beats may interfere with the function of the pacemaker and suppression of such ectopics with lignocaine or some other drug may be required.

Monitoring of permanent pacemakers

Most modern pacemakers are powered with lithium batteries which will function satisfactorily for 5 to 10 years, the life being reduced if a high output or fast rate is required. A regular check on the rate of the pacemaker is routine because, before the pacemaker fails, it goes through a period of gradual decline in rate. Detection of this decline allows routine replacement of the pacemaker unit before failure occurs.

Failure to pace may be due to *malposition* of the catheter electrode. The pervenous catheter can dislodge from the right ventricular endocardium or it can penetrate the wall of the heart. A routine chest x-ray will detect this. *Exit block* may also develop. Even if the catheter remains in good position the myocardial cells in proximity to it fail to transmit the pacing impulse satisfactorily. This may be overcome by increasing the output of the pacemaker. This problem seems more common where epicardial wires are used. Sometimes a brief trial of steroids is worthwhile as conduction may improve. Fracture of pacing wires is now exceedingly rare.

Failure to sense may occur with demand pacemakers. This may not in itself be too important as the unit will effectively return to a fixed rate function. Interpretation of muscle movement, small currents set up by stray unused wires, or other artefacts, as QRS complexes may be a problem if a demand unit fails to pace. High powered radio frequency transmission can also *inhibit* such pacemakers. These include equipment used in arc welding or radio transmitters. Diathermy at operation can also be a problem although this is minimal if the diathermy is below the diaphragm and the indifferent electrode is also lower in the body. If temporary inhibition does occur during operation the pacemaker can be converted to a fixed rate mode by placing a magnet over it. This technique is also used during monitoring of a demand unit if the patient's rate happens to be above the demand rate at the time of observation.

The role of pacemakers has expanded considerably over the last decade so that they now can be used reliably in intermittent block and other intermittent arrhythmias. In the ICU the capacity to maintain the heart rate at optimal level may well prove crucial in a difficult postoperative period. Postoperative pacing is particularly helpful in infants undergoing operation under profound hypothermia and in patients with long standing mitral or multivalve disease, and after tricuspid valve replacement. Atrial pacing is also valuable in the management of supraventricular and ventricular arrhythmias which can often be controlled by pacing at a relatively high rate. Like sinus rhythm, atrial pacing has the advantage that atrial contraction precedes ventricular contraction, and the ventricle is optimally filled before it contracts. If heart block is present, A–V sequential pacing will allow similar control. Temporary pacing wires are attached only loosely to the myocardium and are usually withdrawn 8 to 10 days after operation.

9 Cardiac Intensive Care

NURSING CARE AFTER OPERATIONS ON THE HEART

The goals of intensive care after cardiac surgery can be listed under five headings:

1 Maintenance of stable cardiovascular function and tissue perfusion.
2 Maintenance of respiratory function and adequate oxygenation.
3 Maintenance of fluid, electrolyte and nutritional balance.
4 Support of physical and psychological well being.
5 Recognition and treatment of postoperative complications.

Care of the patient is a team effort — the activities of medical, nursing, physiotherapy, and technical staff are all interdependent. While each speciality has its own function, understanding of overall management is crucial. Particularly in the first 48 hr the patient needs constant assessment, observation and care. A capacity for immediate response to any complication is required as this is the period when most serious problems may arise.

Before operation the patient should have a full understanding of the procedure and management of ICU. Ideally the nursing staff will already know him or her; certainly the nurse will have a full understanding of the patient's medical status and of the social background of both the patient and the relatives who will be supporting him. The parents of infants and children will already have visited the ICU and all visitors should be prepared for the sight of their relative surrounded by apparatus and with endotracheal and drainage tubes in place. At the first opportunity a full explanation of the patient's status and management will be made to the relative, and support of the family will remain an integral part of management throughout the patient's stay.

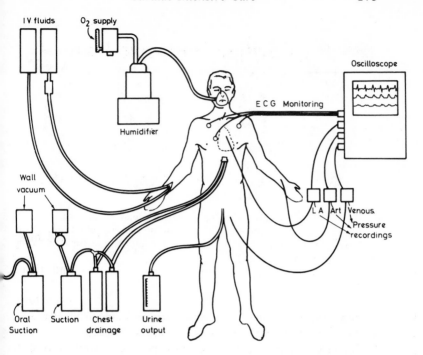

Fig. 50 Intensive care monitoring.

Initial procedures on receiving the patient from the operating theatre

The patient is transferred directly from the operating theatre to the ICU where routine initial observations and procedures are carried out in a systematic fashion to allow an assessment of his or her condition and to provide a baseline for continuing evaluation. These are:

1 Assessment of the patient's colour, level of consciousness and restlessness. Ventilatory status, airway, oxygen mask and oxygen flow rate are checked. If artificial ventilation is required this is established (p. 250).

2 ECG monitoring is begun (Fig. 51). Positioning of the positive and negative electrodes as in Fig. 51a gives a tracing similar to lead II; the arrangement in 51b is MCL_1, similar to lead V_1. Both are satisfactory for monitoring rhythm. Sometimes a lead like V_5 is

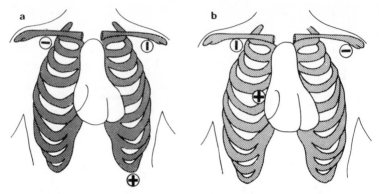

Fig. 51 (a) Lead positions giving a tracing like lead 2; the positive lead is on the left lower chest, the negative lead on the right upper chest; and the indifferent lead on the left upper chest; (b) lead positions for monitoring MCL₁ Conventions as in (a).

useful and this is obtained by shifting the positive electrode to the V_5 position. A rhythm strip is taken for baseline assessment.

3 Suitably identified pressure catheters (right atrial or central venous, arterial, left atrial and sometimes pulmonary arterial) are connected to transducers and continuous pressure monitoring is begun.

4 Drainage tubes, clamped in transit, are connected to underwater seals (Fig. 52). The amount of drainage is noted.

5 Intravenous fluids and blood transfusion are commenced (or continued).

6 The urinary catheter, if present, is joined to its drainage bottle.

7 Core temperature and peripheral temperatures are assessed.

8 Baseline entries are recorded on a flow sheet, such as the example shown in Fig. 53. The flow sheet enables easy assessment of the patient's progress.

Observations and measurements should be recorded at half-hourly intervals, bearing in mind that more frequent records are needed in changing situations and that emergency treatment takes precedence over records.

The bedside observation and careful assessment of the state of consciousness, restlessness, pain, sweating and pallor are as important as the more complicated monitoring procedures.

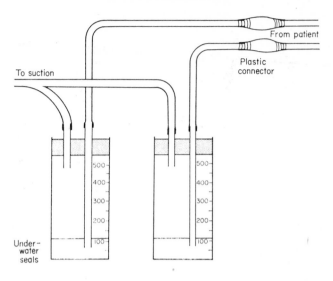

Fig. 52 Diagram to show the arrangement for underwater drainage.

Routine investigations

The following investigations are made as part of the evaluation of the patient's status:

1 Blood: haemoglobin, blood gases, pH, serum electrolytes, plasma haemoglobin, heparin content and clotting time.

2 Chest x-ray: after return from theatre and daily until drainage tubes are removed.

1 Maintenance of stable cardiovascular function and tissue perfusion

Cardiac monitoring (see also p. 229)

Some indication of cardiac output can be obtained from the colour and temperature of the periphery, and from the briskness of flushing after pressure. These signs should be assessed regularly. Monitoring of heart rate and pressures is carried out continuously.

Time	pH	P_{CO_2} mmHg	BASE EXCESS	P_{O_2} mmHg	O₂ Satn %	K+ mmol /l	Hb g/l	Haemo-lysis mg/l	Heparin units/ ml	Clotting time minutes	
1315	7.31	42	−5.1	130	98	3.9	102	321	0.5 or less	7	SURGEON:
1515	7.42	37	−3.5	115	97	4.6	111	230	0.5 or less	5	OPERATION:

CUMULATIVE TOTALS — BLOOD AND PLASMA

DATE & TIME	I	II	III	IV	Total	Lab Amt	Lab Total	TOTAL OUT	PLASMA Level	PLASMA Total given	BLOOD Level	BLOOD Total given	TOTAL IN	BALANCE	URINE Amt	URINE Total
1·8·81																
1210	100	40									700				0	
30	140	50			50			50	500		850	150	150	+100	180	180
13	160	50			20	5	5	75	450	50	875	25	225	+150	150/50	330
30	180	55			25		5	100	400	50	875	−	275	+175	120/20	450
14	190	55			10		5	110	400	−	900	25	300	+190	60/60	510
30	195	60			10		5	120	400	−	925	25	325	+205	25/25	535
15	205	60			10	3	8	133	300	100	925	−	425	+292	30/30	565
30	215	65			15		8	148	250	50	1000	75	550	+402	25/25	590
16	230	65			15		8	163	200	50	500	−	600	+437	20/20	610

Fig. 53 Record-sheet of a patient in the ICU.

Heart rate

Sinus tachycardia, up to 120 per min, may occur after operation. A higher heart rate may be due to pain, anxiety or fever. It may be a response to a low cardiac output due to bleeding or some other cause (p. 147), or be due to an arrhythmia, most often atrial fibrillation or supraventricular tachycardia. In atrioventricular block during the postoperative period the ventricular rate is often high (up to 110 per min); the rate falls, sometimes abruptly, during the first 3 days, to below 60 per min. Sinus bradycardia may occur as a response to preoperative administration of beta blocking agents or to the intraoperative use of cold cardioplegic solution.

If an abrupt change in rate occurs a record should be made and some intervention will probably be required.

Recording and interpretation of intravascular pressures

Care of the transducer. A 'transducer' converts one kind of energy

DATE: 1·8·81	Surname SMITH		MR	11	401	C2244	

MR. KERR

TRIPLE CORONARY VEIN GRAFT

Christian names JOHN HENRY M 28·1·25 56 Auckland

Address 20 South Road, GREENLANE. Dom. Code

Clinical team DR GREEN

FLUID REQUIREMENT: _____
65 ml 5% DEXTROSE Hrly IV

HEIGHT: 170·5 cm
WEIGHT: 64·1 Kg

REMARKS

O₂ by M.C. mask at 4 litres

DAILY TOTALS – FLUIDS									PRESSURES					Minute volume/Tidal volume	Oxygen	Suction	Cuff release		
INPUT																			
Electro-man		I V drip		I V drip		ORAL		TOTAL IN											
Level	Total given	Level	Total given	Level	Total given	Amt	Total given		B P	V P	A B	Resp						
240	70								¹¹⁰/₇₀	7	94	16		✓				KCL 20 mmol
240		50	20				20	20	¹²⁰/₈₀	9	80	16		✓				T 35·6°C FEET COOL
260	20	25	45					65	¹¹⁰/₈₀	8	90	18		✓				SINUS RHYTHM
260	20	0/₇₀	70					90	¹²⁵/₈₀	9	84	18		✓				KCL 20 mmol
280	40	50	90					130	¹²⁰/₈₀	9	80	20		✓				PAPAVERETUM 5 mg IV
280	40	20	120					160	¹¹⁰/₈₀	8	94	18		✓				
300	60	0/₇₀	140					200	¹²⁰/₈₀	9	80	20		✓				
300	60	40	170					230	¹²⁵/₈₀	9	84	20		✓				T 36·5°C
300	60	10	200					260	¹¹⁵/₈₀	8	86	20		✓				

into another — in this case mechanical energy (pressure) into electrical energy. The electrical signal is then amplified and displayed on an oscilloscope and/or pen-recorder. The transducer is delicate and expensive and must be handled with care. Regular calibration is

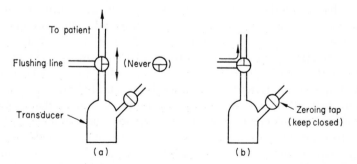

To patient

Flushing line ═══ (Never ⊖)

Transducer

Zeroing tap (keep closed)

(a) (b)

Fig. 54 Tap-positions for (a) pressure-recording and (b) for flushing pressure-lines.

required and an arterial pressure-trace can be quickly and frequently checked by comparing it with an ordinary cuff measurement. Blood should never be allowed to enter a transducer, nor should the transducer be exposed to the high pressure generated by flushing; the appropriate tap positions are shown in Fig. 54.

Care of the pressure lines. Pressure lines should be kept patent at all times. Obstruction or kinking of the lines leads to damping or disappearance of the pressure trace; the lines should be flushed with a heparinised intravenous solution. Some Units prefer to use a constant slow infusion to aid in maintenance of patency of pressure lines. Bleeding at the site of insertion of a catheter is usually readily controlled by local manual pressure.

Measurement of pressure is made from a defined 'zero' level and the pressures recorded will thus depend on the choice of zero, the pressure being higher if the zero is lower and vice versa. A satisfactory zero level is the mid-thoracic position at the 4th intercostal space. Transducers must be adjusted to this with a spirit level. This compensates fairly well for the changes in the patient's position if he lies on his back, but there is no satisfactory zero level for a patient lying on his side.

  The *filling pressure* of the heart, being much lower than arterial pressure, is relatively more dependent on the zero level. From the midthoracic position normal right atrial or central venous pressure is about 5 mmHg and left atrial pressure is 5 mmHg higher. When left sided failure is present, however, left atrial pressure can be as much as 20 mmHg higher than right atrial pressure. Optimal filling is required to achieve the best cardiac output and, in the presence of left sided failure, a left atrial pressure of 15 to 20 mmHg may be required (though not usually more than 10 to 12 mmHg in infants). Similarly a right ventricular filling pressure of 10 to 12 mmHg may be required when right-sided failure is present. Falling atrial pressure in the presence of low cardiac output indicates inadequate volume replacement, and rising pressure may indicate overtransfusion, failure of the ventricle concerned, or tamponade. Management is aimed at achieving a filling pressure prescribed for the individual patient. During replacement of blood loss, the stage of optimal correction is seen when the venous pressure is significantly raised by a small increase in blood or other volume expander (100 ml in an adult).

A fall in arterial pressure may mean:

1 *Uncorrected blood loss.* Because of compensation (p. 63), much blood may be lost before arterial pressure falls. Filling pressure falls much sooner and is a more sensitive guide to the need for transfusion.

2 *A severe fall in cardiac output,* despite an adequate venous pressure. This is due to cardiac failure or tamponade and calls for urgent treatment (p. 189). Since venous pressure is not reduced, transfusion does not help and may overload the heart still further.

Volume replacement

It is almost always necessary to transfuse more volume than the measured loss, partly because some of the shed blood remains in the chest and partly because some vascular beds are still dilating after operation. Postoperatively the patient is usually transfused to a venous or right atrial pressure of about 10 to 12 mmHg and a left atrial pressure of about 15 mmHg. If cardiac output is satisfactory these pressures are allowed to fall gradually but, if output is low, the pressures are maintained. If left ventricular function is the main problem, e.g. after mitral or aortic valve surgery, adequacy of blood volume replacement is judged by left atrial pressure. If right ventricular function is the main problem, e.g. after correction of tetralogy of Fallot, adequacy of replacement is judged by right atrial pressure. Inability to maintain adequate arterial pressure indicates a failing ventricle or continued bleeding and requires urgent intervention. Infants and children seldom need a venous pressure above 7 mmHg or a left atrial pressure above 10 mmHg.

The choice of volume expander varies. Blood removed at operation is replaced but additional blood products are given only if required. Although a low haemoglobin limits the oxygen carrying capacity of blood many patients cope perfectly well with a haemoglobin of about 100 g per l. For a patient with a critically low cardiac output, however, an optimal haemoglobin is essential. If transfusion is required packed red blood cells are best used. For pure volume expansion a blood substitute such as haemaccel, dextran or stable plasma protein solution (p. 11) may be used. Freeze dried plasma protein or fresh blood may be required if haemostasis is a problem.

The urinary output

With a *clear prime* a diuresis is usual during and immediately after bypass. Urinary output then falls but should not drop below 20 ml per hr; lower values usually indicate a low cardiac output. Flows should gradually increase to average over 0·5 ml per kg per hr over the 24 hr period. With a *blood prime* the early diuresis is less marked and the patient should maintain a relatively steady urine output throughout. Persistent oliguria is a valuable index of a low cardiac output, provided that dehydration and renal disease can be excluded. An increasing urinary flow soon follows improvement in cardiac output. The volume of urine should therefore be recorded half-hourly. Other losses, such as gastric aspirate, are of course similarly recorded.

A urinary catheter is required after use of a clear prime because of the resultant diuresis. If cardiac output is low continued catheterisation is scarcely avoidable, since the valuable information given by measurement of urinary flow usually outweighs the risk of infection. This risk demands the removal of the catheter as soon as possible.

2   Maintenance of respiratory function and adequate oxygenation

Continuous assessment of the patient's respiratory status is essential. Assessment includes observation of the patient's colour and blood gas analysis is undertaken at intervals. Details of respiratory care are given in Chapter 11.

Deep breathing exercises and regular turning of the patient are begun once his or her cardiovascular status is stable, to encourage chest expansion and prevent pooling of secretions and atelectasis.

Drainage tubes

There will usually be two pericardial drainage tubes, so placed in order to avoid the accumulation of blood in the mediastinum. Extra drainage tubes are placed in the pleural cavity if the pleura has been opened. Each is connected to an *underwater-seal* (Fig. 52) so that air cannot pass along the tube into the chest. Mediastinal tubes are not stitched in place and can be shortened as needed merely by pulling on them. The bung must fit tightly into the drainage vessel, and *the drainage tube must connect with the long tube which dips below the surface of the sterile water.* The short tube which ends just below the bung can be joined to a wall suction line to assist in drainage. The volume and appearance of drainage fluid are recorded. Absence of drainage may mean that the tube is blocked. To ensure that drainage tubes are patent they must be milked frequently and kinking must be prevented. If the drainage tube is blocked it may need to be withdrawn a little or the obstruction removed. Drainage greater than 100 ml per half-hour indicates excessive bleeding and usually requires additional steps.

All being well, the tubes can be removed the day after operation but, if an atrial catheter is required for a longer period, one tube is usually left in place in case bleeding should follow removal of the catheter. The management of pleural drains is described on p. 267.

3   Maintenance of fluid, electrolyte and nutritional balance

Water and electrolyte balance

Intravenous replacement must avoid dehydration (viscid secretions and oliguria) and overhydration (cardiac failure and pulmonary oedema). After operation, renal excretion of sodium and water is impaired and less replacement is needed during the first day.

Water. The minimal requirement is 700 to 800 ml per m² body surface area per 24 hr for the first 2 days. This amounts to 30 ml per m² per hr. In an adult this works out at something in the region of 1 ml per kg per hr but in a baby it is closer to 2 ml per kg per hr. More will be needed in the presence of fever, gastric suction or established dehydration.

Sodium. After a cardiac operation sodium depletion is rare; total body sodium is almost always increased and sodium excretion is reduced. Sodium is not usually needed for 48 hr and during the following 2 to 3 days 25 mmol per m² per day (40 mmol in the average adult) is usually enough. The serum Na^+ concentration is usually no guide whatever to requirements. A low serum Na^+ is usually due to overhydration or to an abnormal exchange of Na^+ and K^+ between cells and extracellular fluid (p. 10); the corresponding treatment is therefore water restriction or potassium repletion. The presence of oedema almost always guarantees that the body content of sodium is increased.

Potassium. The serum K^+ concentration is a poor guide to the body content of K^+, and in K^+ depletion is more often normal than reduced; most of the body K^+ is in the cells. Potassium loss and a falling serum K^+ are usual postoperatively, especially in patients given diuretics previously. This depletion promotes arrhythmias, especially when digitalis is given. Intravenous potassium, up to 20 mmol per hr, offsets this tendency. The adult requirement of K^+ is about 40 mmol per day unless the above special circumstances arise; a good deal more may be required during the first postoperative day.

Other electrolytes. Calcium is sometimes needed if a lot of citrated blood has been given. Citrate can produce alkalosis which increases urinary loss of potassium.

Management of fluid replacement

The needs previously mentioned can be supplied by appropriate combinations of the following standard solutions:
1   *1/5 isotonic saline plus 4·2 per cent glucose:* 30 mmol Na^+, 42 g glucose per l.
2   *Isotonic saline:* 150 mmol Na^+ per l. This is rarely used.
3   5 per cent glucose: 50 g glucose per l.
4   *Potassium chloride solution,* for addition to infusion bottles, KCL is made up in ampoules containing either 10 mmol of K^+ or 1 g of KCL (equal to 13 mmol of K^+) in 10 ml of water.

During the first 24 to 48 hr fluid requirements are generally given as 5 per cent glucose, with potassium supplements as indicated. Thereafter two-thirds of the requirement is given as one-fifth isotonic saline plus 4·2 per cent glucose, and the other one-third as 5 per cent glucose.

Intravenous infusions, fluid used to flush the catheters and any water given orally are recorded half-hourly, and included in the 24-hr intake.

Nutrition

Feeding is not required during the first 24 hr but must be considered after 48 hr because inadequate supply of calories will lead to excessive catabolism of body protein with muscle wasting and poor wound healing. After uncomplicated cardiac or thoracic surgery, oral fluids may be started on the first postoperative day. When bowel sounds and the passage of flatus are established a light diet is introduced and should supply the estimated daily protein and calorie requirements (Appendix 3). If the patient cannot eat, the normal diet can be homogenized and given through a nasogastric tube. Homogenized feeds are easy to make up and are relatively cheap, but there is always some uncertainty about the exact content of the diet and a risk of bacterial contamination during preparation. A synthetic diet such as Thrive or Complan has a known composition with all the essential nutrients (Appendix 3).

Nasogastric feeding may cause diarrhoea particularly if milk or milk products are included. This problem can sometimes be overcome by the use of one of the elemental diets like Vivonex or Flexical which require no digestion. These products are expensive but are used commonly during management of multiple malabsorption states and fistulae of the gastrointestinal tract.

When a patient is unable to take oral or nasogastric tube feeds, protein and calories must be given intravenously. This technique is called *total parenteral nutrition,* and entails the infusion of:

1 An amino acid preparation (e.g. aminofusin, freamine, amigen) which supplies the building blocks for protein synthesis. These solutions contain the equivalent of 50 to 100 gm of protein per litre.

2 Glucose 25 to 50 per cent solution; 50 per cent glucose provides 2000 Calories per litre.

Solutions 1 and 2 are both hypertonic and if given rapidly can lead to cellular dehydration from osmotic action (p. 8). They are also irritants and are usually administered via a central vein.

3 A fat emulsion (e.g. intralipid 10 to 20 per cent fat). A 20 per cent emulsion supplies 2000 Calories per litre. The preparation is not irritant and behaves osmotically like plasma. However, the emulsion can easily be precipitated and for this reason it should not be shaken or mixed with saline. It is stored at 4°C. If given too rapidly side effects may occur abruptly. These are pyrexia and breathlessness.

4 Electrolyte solutions to give the calculated requirement of Na^+, K^+, Ca^{2+}, Mg^{2+} and PO_4^{3-}.

The requirements of an individual patient can be met by varying the volume of concentration of any of the above infusions.

The infusions are given through a central venous cannula and begun slowly, the total requirements not being met for several days.

It is important that the infusions run at a constant rate throughout each 24 hr period to avoid large swings in blood glucose concentrations. If glucose appears in the urine it indicates that endogenous insulin secretion is insufficient and insulin should be added to the infusion or given according to a sliding scale. A dual-connection can be used to allow the simultaneous infusion of two preparations provided it is remembered that intralipid and saline are not compatible and that a source of calories should always be infused with the amino acid solutions to prevent the latter being metabolised to produce energy.

A regimen which provides 125 gm of protein and 3500 Calories (14·7 kJ) together with electrolytes is described in Appendix 3. A multivitamin injection and 1 mg of folic acid are given daily while Vitamin K 10 mg weekly and Vitamin B_{12} as required are given intramuscularly. Trace elements are added if the therapy is prolonged. Additional calories can be supplied by the infusion of intralipid 10 or 20 per cent, but even if the calories are not required 500 ml should be given twice weekly to supply essential fatty acids.

Blood pressure, heart rate and respiratory frequency should be carefully monitored especially when the infusion is started, and accurate balance sheets kept. Twenty-four hr collections of urine are made for estimations of sodium, potassium and urea, and urinary glucose is estimated 4-hourly. Blood urea, electrolytes and glucose concentration are measured daily and the composition of the infusion changed if necessary. The volume and composition may also have to be altered in the presence of certain diseases. For example, cardiac failure may necessitate volume restriction while solutions used in renal failure contain only essential amino acids.

Infection is a serious hazard of total parenteral nutrition since the preparations used favour the rapid multiplication of bacteria. The administration sets and connections should be changed aseptically every 24 hrs. At 48 hr intervals the catheterization site should be inspected, cleaned with Tincture of Iodine and redressed with an air occlusive dressing after applying Povidone Iodine ointment. The central catheter should be used for the total parenteral nutrition only and other routes for the administration of drugs and blood transfusions.

4 Support of physical and psychological well-being

Maintenance of body temperature

Pyrexia often occurs for a few days (p. 28). A temperature exceeding 39°C is extra stress and cooling by fan, stripping of bedclothes to a single sheet, or even tepid sponging may be needed. Aspirin (0·3 to 0·6 g) or paracetamol (0·5 to 1 g) help to reduce fever. If persistent, an infective cause should be sought.

Promotion of movement

Regular active and passive movements of all limbs, correct positioning and regular position changes prevent complications associated with immobility.

Promotion of rest, comfort, relief from pain

Restlessness is commonly due to pain or a full bladder, but hypoxia, bleeding or a low cardiac output must always be thought of and treated if present. Otherwise papaveretum or diazepam, both 5 to 10 mg IV may be given, papaveretum being preferred if pain is important.

Regular attention to pressure areas, frequent position changes, the avoidance of uncomfortable positions, regular mouth care, the grouping of nursing procedures to avoid disturbing the patient unnecessarily all contribute to minimising patient discomfort.

Assessment of neurological function

The patient's level of consciousness, pupillary response, ability to move all limbs, and orientation are all assessed in the immediate postoperative period and kept under scrutiny thereafter.

5 Recognition and treatment of postoperative complications

Minimizing mental confusion, anxiety, fear and tension are important aspects of care. Preoperative teaching and explanatory sessions both to patients and their families are indispensable. Carefully prescribed pain relief, allowing as much privacy and rest as possible, and encouraging free contact with immediate family all contribute. The patient should be reassured about his or her progress and have procedures fully explained. Above all the patient must be recognized at all times as an individual who is under particular stress and has special needs.

RECOGNITION AND TREATMENT OF POSTOPERATIVE COMPLICATIONS

Bleeding

Copious bleeding is usually evident from the drained volume, but quite often drainage is incomplete. The nurse must thus be alert for other signs — tachycardia, restlessness, and fall in venous, left atrial (and later arterial) pressure. When these signs are out of proportion to the amount of blood drained, a chest x-ray may show an undrained accumulation. Partial withdrawal of the drainage tube or changing of the patient's position may promote drainage. Continued bleeding requires surgical exploration to identify and stop it. The 'acceptable' loss of blood, before exploration becomes necessary, depends on the size of the patient. An infant's blood volume is 80 to 100 ml per kg, and a loss of 60 ml in a 3 kg baby is 20 per cent of the blood volume — a serious haemorrhage.

Defects in the clotting mechanism. Arrest of bleeding from the field of operation demands that the clotting mechanism be unimpaired. A clot is a web of *fibrin,* a protein, containing blood cells in its meshes. Fibrin is formed from a precursor, *fibrinogen,* one of the normal plasma proteins, by the action of another protein, thrombin. The precursor of thrombin is *prothrombin.* Many other substances, including *calcium,* and *platelets* are essential for normal clotting to occur. The following abnormalities of the clotting mechanism may cause prolonged bleeding.

1 *Heparin* is an anticoagulant because it interferes with the formation and action of thrombin. It is routinely administered before bypass is begun and its effect is later neutralized by the injection of protamine. Neutralization is sometimes incomplete and extra protamine may be needed postoperatively.

2 *Anticoagulants* acting at other points in the clotting process may

appear in the circulating blood, for obscure reasons, from time to time. An excess of protamine, paradoxically, may act as an anti-coagulant.

3 Platelet deficiency (*thrombocytopenia*) is not uncommon. It may result from the consumption of platelets during intravascular coagulation (see below) but has many other possible causes. If responsible for bleeding it may be treated by infusion of fresh blood or platelet concentrate.

4 *Prothrombin deficiency* is found in severe liver disease, as after prolonged hepatic congestion. Freeze-dried plasma supplies pro-thrombin and other essential clotting factors. Vitamin K, a precur-sor of prothrombin, may be given by injection.

5 *Calcium deficiency.* Large transfusions of stored, citrated blood may deplete ionized calcium, and calcium chloride or gluconate should be given to forestall this. Serum total calcium estimations will not reveal a deficiency of ionized calcium.

6 *Disseminated intravascular coagulation.* States of low cardiac output, especially with septicaemia, are sometimes complicated by the occurrence of widespread clotting in the smallest arteries and veins. This has two results. First, the peripheral circulation is still further slowed. Secondly, clotting factors are used up and are not available to help stop bleeding at some other site. Typically, platelet count and fibrinogen content of the blood are reduced. Paradoxi-cally, treatment consists in giving heparin to prevent the small-vessel clotting, together with transfusion of fresh blood to provide platelets, fibrinogen and other factors.

7 *Stored blood* is deficient in clotting factors, and a bleeding tendency may arise when large transfusions have been necessary. Freeze-dried plasma or fresh blood supply the needed factors.

Cardiac tamponade

A collection of blood in the pericardium restricts the filling of the heart and cardiac output falls. The typical signs of tamponade are (1) rising venous pressure; (2) falling arterial pressure; (3) pulsus paradoxus — the systolic pressure is higher, by more than 10 mmHg, during expiration than during inspiration; the converse is the case if the patient is being ventilated by respirator.

Arterial pressure is normally slightly higher in expiration but this is exaggerated in the presence of tamponade. With the fall in intrathoracic pressure on inspiration, pulmonary venous return is inhibited by the distended pericardium, left ventricular output falls transiently and arterial pressure drops. With positive pressure ventilation the pressure situation is reversed; intrathoracic pressure is higher in inspiration so that left-ventricular filling is better and arterial pressure higher; (4) The chest x-ray shows an increase in the cardiac shadow.

Unless adequate drainage from the pericardium can be restored by shortening pericardial drains, surgical exploration is essential. The possibility of tamponade must be kept constantly in mind, since even mild tamponade is a fairly common contributory cause of low cardiac output.

Low cardiac output

The normal resting cardiac output is 3 l per min per square metre (m^2) of body surface area, or about 5 l per min in an average adult of $1 \cdot 7 \ m^2$. Immediately after a cardiac operation the output is usually normal but it may fall after 12 to 24 hr to levels of 2 l per min per m^2 or even lower, depending on the severity of the disease and the extent of the operation. A very low output is dangerous and its measurement in the ICU is a valuable guide to correct treatment.

Measurement of cardiac output. In the ICU, cardiac output is most easily measured by an indicator dilution method.

If 1 mg of an indicator substance is mixed thoroughly with an unknown volume of blood in a beaker (Fig. 55) and the resulting concentration of indicator is found to be $0 \cdot 5$ mg per l, the volume of blood must obviously have been 2 l. The calculation is thus:

$$\text{Volume of blood} = \frac{\text{Amount of indicator}}{\text{Concentration of indicator}} = \frac{1 \text{ mg}}{0 \cdot 5 \text{ mg per l}} = 2 \text{ l}$$

This principle is used in the measurement of cardiac output, but since the volume measured is the amount of blood flowing in a given time the calculation is a little more complex. For example, if an indicator dye is injected into the pulmonary artery it is diluted in the volume of blood which sweeps it through the lungs and its concentration can be measured continuously as it appears in the aorta or a peripheral artery (Fig. 55). Then:

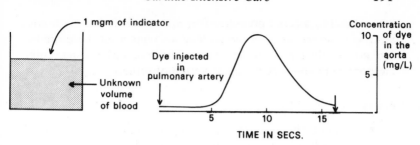

Fig. 55 (a) Principle of indicator dye dilution. (b) Dye dilution curve.

$$\frac{\text{Cardiac}}{\text{output}} = \frac{\text{Amount of dye injected}}{\text{(Mean concentration of the dye during inscription of dye curve)} \times \text{Duration of dye curve}}$$

The principle of the thermodilution method is similar. A bolus of cold saline or glucose solution is injected into the right atrium and its concentration in the pulmonary artery deduced from the change in temperature it produces there. The calculation of cardiac output is very like that used for the dye-dilution method.

Causes of low cardiac output. (1) Cardiac failure due to myocardial disease, to valvar or septal abnormalities, or to the effects of surgical trauma. (2) An inadequate blood-volume due either to bleeding or to vasodilatation. (3) Tamponade.

Effects. A change occurs in the normal distribution of blood flow to the body (p. 51). In general, this change ensures that vital regions receive blood at the expense of less vulnerable regions. Flow to the brain, heart and suprarenal glands is well maintained. Flow to the skin, kidneys, and spleen is markedly reduced, and flow to the gut and liver moderately reduced. Flow to muscle is variable, tending at first to fall sharply and then to rise, though not to normal levels. These adjustments are made by selective arteriolar constriction brought about by the baroreceptor reflex (p. 56).

Since the total peripheral vascular resistance (p. 50) is consequently increased, arterial pressure tends to be maintained for a time despite the decline in cardiac output. When, however, the degree of arteriolar constriction approaches its maximum, little additional compensation is possible and a further fall in output will cause a fall in arterial pressure. *This is a relatively late event and signifies a serious drop in output.* Earlier signs must therefore be looked for diligently; these are restlessness, tachycardia, cool, sweating skin and a declining excretion of urine.

Shock

This is a popular but rather vague term, used here to mean a state in which, owing to a reduction in cardiac output, the circulation cannot maintain essential functions. As so defined, shock is almost invariably associated with a fall in arterial pressure. It is marked by the widespread reduction in blood flow already described which, while tolerable for a short time, eventually leads to serious and even irreversible changes which include the following.

1 *Kidneys.* Oliguria, tubular necrosis and uraemia (reversible); renal cortical ischaemia or necrosis (irreversible). Renal impairment is a special hazard in the presence of postoperative protein breakdown and release of potassium into the circulation (p. 25); hyperkalaemia with cardiac arrhythmias is a particular risk in children after correction of cyanotic heart disease.
2 Formation and release of *lactic acid* due to lack of oxygen in the cells. A state of cellular and extracellular acidosis develops. This leads in turn to:
a Diminished cardiac efficiency with a tendency to cardiac arrhythmias.
b Relaxation of arterioles, with further fall in arterial pressure.
c Pooling of blood in the capillaries, leading to reduced venous return and further impairment of cardiac output.
3 *Disseminated intravascular coagulation.*
4 *Myocardial depression.* Inadequate perfusion of the abdominal organs, especially of the pancreas, leads to the formation of a substance known as 'myocardial depressant factor' which impairs myocardial contractility.

A vicious cycle is thus established (Fig. 56), the correction of which becomes progressively more difficult. Sooner or later death ensues from cardiac arrest or brain damage.

Treatment of postoperative shock

1 Tamponade, haemothorax, or other undrained bleeding must

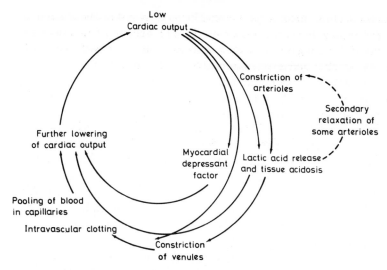

Fig. 56   The vicious cycle in circulatory shock.

be treated as necessary.

2   Blood is infused to ensure adequate filling of the heart, as indicated by a venous pressure of 10 to 15 mmHg, or a left atrial pressure of 15 to 20 mmHg.

3   Adequate ventilation must be ensured, usually by respirator (p. 250).

4   Correction of metabolic acidosis by infusion of bicarbonate.

5   Improvement of cardiac function:

a   Rapid digitalization (p. 110).

b   Continuous infusion of isoprenaline or other inotropic agent (p. 117).

c   Intravenous calcium chloride *except when serum potassium is reduced.*

d   Regulation of ventricular rate by pacemaker if necessary (p. 165). Atrial pacemaker wires are often inserted at operation for this purpose.

6   Treatment directed towards the peripheral circulation (Fig. 57).

The effects of vasodilatation have already been discussed (p. 118) and are illustrated in Fig. 57a. Intravenous nitroglycerine will reduce left ventricular end diastolic pressure and thereby reduce pulmonary venous congestion; it also dilates the coronary arteries.

Its effect on cardiac index is usually modest and extreme caution is required with its usage in patients who are already hypotensive. Sodium nitroprusside, with its potent effect on preload and after-load is often preferred where the primary problem is low cardiac output. In practice in the ICU, an inotropic agent is usually already in use when vasodilator therapy is considered. As shown in Fig. 57b, inotropic agents increase cardiac index but have little direct effect on preload. An increase in cardiac index may, of course, allow the systemic vascular resistance to fall; the heart is then working against a lower afterload and the LVED pressure may fall secondar-ily. In this case the inotrope alone is enough. When this does not occur, improved cardiac index and lowered LVED pressure may be achieved by the addition of a vasodilator as shown in Fig. 57b.

For convenience the administration of inotropic agents and vas-odilators has been discussed in the management of shock. It is self evident, however, that the best results will be achieved when low cardiac output is recognized and treated at any early stage.

7   *Intra-aortic balloon pumping.* Counter pulsation by an intra-aortic balloon pump reduces the afterload of the left ventricle and improves coronary arterial blood flow. A large balloon catheter is introduced under sterile conditions into the femoral artery and is advanced to the descending thoracic aorta. Using an ECG trigger, the balloon inflates in early diastole, sequential inflation of the small distal segment and the larger proximal segment ensuring that blood is forced back towards the coronary arteries and that proxi-mal aortic pressure is maintained (Fig. 58). In early systole the balloon deflates, pressure drops markedly in the ascending aorta and the afterload of the left ventricle is thereby diminished. The workload of the ventricle may be reduced by 40 per cent and the coronary flow increased by 20 per cent. The benefits of this proce-dure are further illustrated in Fig. 59. The left ventricle performs work by pumping blood against arterial pressure. The product of the systolic pressure and the duration of systole gives a measure of this work; in Fig. 59 this is represented by the shaded area labelled SPTI, the systolic pressure-time index. This index gives a measure of the oxygen requirement of the ventricle and hence its require-ment for coronary blood flow. Eighty per cent of coronary blood flow occurs in diastole and it is dependent on the difference in diastolic pressures in the aorta and the left ventricle. A measure of coronary blood flow is therefore given by the shaded area in diastole

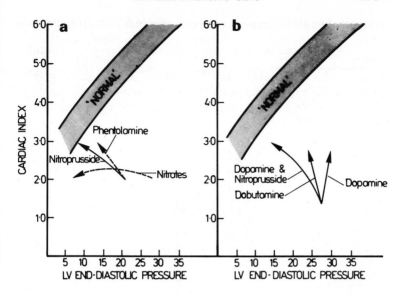

Fig. 57 Diagramatic representation of the relationship between LV filling pressure and cardiac output. As LVED pressure increases so does the cardiac output (Starling's Law). The 'NORMAL' range shows the response of the heart to infusion of fluids. Under normal circumstances the relationship between LVED pressure and cardiac index depends on the contractile state of the myocardium, largely determined by autonomic tone. With exercise for example, the rise in cardiac index with an increase in LVED pressure from 5 to 20 mmHg is much greater than that shown. (a) Nitrates dilate veins with little effect on arterioles (Table 12, p. 123); LVED pressure (the preload) falls with little change in cardiac index. Phentolamine dilates arterioles (i.e. lowers the afterload) with little effect on veins. Cardiac index rises and, because the afterload of the ventricle is lessened, LVED pressure actually falls. Sodium nitroprusside affects both veins and arterioles and its response curve therefore has an intermediate position. (b) Note that the starting point shows a more severe depression of cardiac function than that shown in (a). Dopamine and dobutamine in moderate doses improve cardiac index; because there is only modest effect on veins or arterioles there is little effect on filling pressures. (The effect of digoxin is similar). Adding nitroprusside to one of these drugs lowers both preload and afterload and thereby simultaneously raises cardiac index further while it lowers filling pressure.

labelled DPTI, the diastolic pressure-time index. Clearly the ratio $\frac{DPTI}{SPTI}$ gives a measure of coronary blood flow $\frac{supply}{demand}$. A ventricle will fail if this ratio falls much below 0·7. Fig. 59 shows graphically how the ratio is increased by balloon counter pulsation. (The same principle applies to the reduction of preload and afterload by vasodilator drugs).

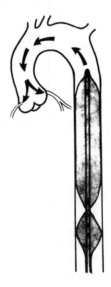

Fig. 58 Diagram of the inflated intra-aortic balloon. Inflation in early diastole raises the pressure in the ascending aorta and forces blood toward the coronaries. The balloon deflates in early systole.

The balloon is filled with carbon dioxide and is connected to an external balloon enclosed in a perspex chamber. Applying a vacuum to the chamber deflates the intra-aortic balloon, and releasing the vacuum reinflates it. A number of problems may arise in the use of the intra-aortic balloon.

1 Gas leaks occur in the system and carbon dioxide must be replaced.

2 The timing of inflation and deflation is critical. A change in heart rate of 20 beats per min will seriously interfere with the function of

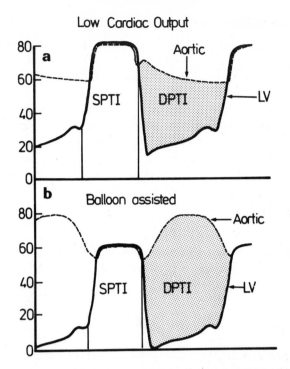

Fig. 59 (a) LV, AO and LA pressures in a failing ventricle and (b) the same pressures when balloon counter pulsation is introduced. The ratio DPTI/SPTI gives an indication of coronary arterial $\dfrac{\text{Supply}}{\text{Demand}}$ (see text). Note the striking improvement in the ratio when balloon counter pulsation is introduced.

the balloon and the effects of rapid atrial fibrillation or frequent ventricular premature beats are even worse.

3 The circulation to the limb through which the catheter has been inserted may become impaired.

Complete familiarity with the equipment is obviously essential for its safe use. Other means of supporting the failing ventricle are continued and meticulous recording of all cardiovascular variables is maintained. In weaning the patient from the balloon catheter, counter pulsation may be applied every 2nd, 3rd or 4th beat.

Pulmonary oedema

This, like cardiac oedema elsewhere, is due to a raised venous and capillary pressure, which forces fluid out of the capillaries into the interstitial fluid. Occurring in the lungs, oedema is an immediate danger.

During the early postoperative period it may be due to pre-existing heart disease with the added handicap of surgical trauma; or it may arise from a fresh myocardial infarct which especially older patients may develop in the first few days, occasionally as a result of coronary embolism during operation. Excessive infusion of blood, plasma or saline predisposes to the development of pulmonary oedema.

The earliest sign is dyspnoea with rapid, shallow breathing and increasing anxiety. Tachycardia, sweating and coldness of the skin follow. Frothy sputum, sometimes pink from bloodstaining, may be produced. Finally cyanosis is added to the pallor. All these signs may develop very rapidly.

Treatment

1 Morphine, 5 to 20 mg intravenously, acts by relieving distress, by vasodilatation, and possibly by other means.
2 Frusemide, 20 to 40 mg intravenously, may cause an immediate diuresis but is not always effective in the early postoperative period.
3 Intravenous infusions are stopped.
4 Digoxin and isoprenaline or some other inotrope are given to improve left ventricular performance.
5 A rapid reduction of LVED pressure may be achieved with intravenous nitroglycerine. An arteriolar vasodilator may also be advantageous; lowering the afterload may reduce LVED pressure.
6 When pulmonary oedema threatens life, tracheal intubation and positive-pressure ventilation may hold it in check while other measures have time to act. The increase in alveolar gas pressure opposes the escape of oedema fluid from the pulmonary capillaries, at the price of reducing cardiac output.
7 Rarely it may be necessary to remove up to 500 ml of blood. This reduces blood volume, venous return and cardiac output, and pressures behind both ventricles fall; the drop in left atrial and pulmonary venous pressure is the object of blood letting.

Congestive cardiac failure

Failure of the right side of the heart dominates the clinical picture, but pulmonary congestion is often present

Features

1 Raised venous pressure.
2 Oedema of the dependent parts, with or without pulmonary congestion.
3 Enlargement of the liver and ascites.
4 Oliguria; the kidneys retain Na^+ and water due in part to (a) reduced renal blood flow, (b) renal congestion and (c) aldosterone secretion (p. 24).
5 Often the serum Na^+ is reduced. Despite this, body sodium content is nearly always high, because (a) the extracellular volume (p. 10) is increased and (b) cellular sodium is increased. The persistence of a low serum (and thus extracellular) sodium concentration, and therefore a low osmolality (p. 93) is due to excessive secretion of antidiuretic hormone (p. 12) with resulting impairment of water excretion.
6 Serum K^+ is usually normal, but total body K^+ (which lies mostly in the cells) is very often reduced, sometimes grossly.

Treatment

1 Digitalis (p. 109).
2 Diuretics (p. 107); thiazides or frusemide are most often used. Spironolactone or amiloride are reserved for the more resistant cases.
3 Sodium restriction (to 40 mmol per day), modest fluid restriction and potassium supplements (50 mmol per day orally).
4 Vasodilators (p. 118) are added in difficult cases.

Arrhythmias (p. 141)

These are very common and hazardous postoperative complications. They are precipitated and aggravated by hypoxia, low cardiac output, potassium depletion, metabolic acidosis and injudicious administration of digitalis. The more dangerous ventricular arrhythmias are most often seen with severe valve lesions and a long history of cardiac failure, and in patients with complicating coronary disease. Postoperative atrioventricular block seldom arises unless block has been present before or during operation.

Any arrhythmia should be recorded; connecting the atrial wire to the V lead of the ECG machine may allow identification in difficult cases. The treatment of arrhythmias has been described (p. 141). In summary, it includes the following:

1 Maintenance of adequate ventilation and of normal blood-gas tensions reduces the liability to arrhythmias.

2 Pacing at an optimal rate can be effective in controlling an arrhythmia. Sometimes frequent supraventricular ectopics, bursts of supraventricular tachycardia, or frequent ventricular ectopics will disappear with atrial pacing at a rate of about 110. When a supraventricular tachycardia is present, a brief period of overdrive pacing at a rate of about 150 per min may achieve capture and abolish the arrhythmia; a more normal pacing rate can then be resumed.

3 Quinidine type drugs which depress the myocardium must be used with caution and beta blocking drugs are usually avoided. If supraventricular tachycardia can not be controlled with digitalis or pacing, DC cardioversion is usually indicated. Intravenous disopyramide is effective in suppressing recurrent supraventricular arrhythmias.

4 Frequent ventricular ectopic beats are usually suppressed with lignocaine, procainamide or mexiletine. Rapid ventricular tachycardia or ventricular fibrillation need immediate DC cardioversion.

Cardiac arrest

This means that the heart has stopped beating effectively. Ventricular standstill or asystole is one cause, but ventricular fibrillation and less often ventricular tachycardia may produce the same functional result. Instant action is essential and all staff must be familiar with the steps required.

Recognition of cardiac arrest. (1) A conscious patient suddenly becomes unconscious, or an unconscious patient changes in some way, e.g. the pattern of breathing changes or convulsive movements are seen; (2) pulses are absent; the carotid or femoral pulses are the most easily felt; (3) heart sounds cannot be heard; (4) the pupils dilate; (5) if an ECG trace is being displayed on the oscilloscope, the wave form is characteristic (p. 158) and the arterial pressure trace is flat; other confirmatory signs are unnecessary, and valuable time must not be wasted in looking for them.

Immediate action. (1) Give a precordial thump and call for help. (2) Insert an oral airway and ventilate with mouth-to-mouth breathing or via a mask with an Ambu bag. If the patient already has the trachea intubated, use this tube for ventilation. (3) Start external cardiac massage.

Two nurses are needed, one to give cardiac massage while the other ventilates. Five cardiac compressions and one full breath should be given separately and in sequence. A third nurse, the ICU doctor, and an anaesthetist should be summoned urgently.

Detailed management

1 *Cardiac massage.* Lay the patient flat and put boards transversely under the mattress if they are not already present; cardiac surgical patients should be nursed on beds with boards. Kneel on the bed beside the patient and apply sharp, firm pressure 60 times per min with hands superposed over the sternum, keeping elbows straight and moving from the shoulders. After each compression, release quickly and completely. An oscilloscope trace should show a systolic pressure of 70 to 100 mmHg. If a trace is not available a good femoral pulse should be felt; if not, massage is not adequate and must be modified until it is. Massage must continue until a heartbeat is restored, and is done by two or three people in relay.

For infants, place one hand behind the chest and one in front, and compress the heart between the fingers at 90 per min. Fingerpressure is enough. Be careful not to let the infant cool, as tends to happen quickly.

2 A *full inspiration from the Ambu bag* is given after every 5 cardiac compressions. Do not interrupt the rhythm of massage to ventilate. *Connect the oxygen supply* to the bag as soon as possible.

3 The third nurse meanwhile should *connect ECG leads and record lead II*. If the rhythm is ventricular tachycardia or fibrillation,

DC cardioversion (p. 115) is tried at once. If asytole, drugs are given (see below). Cardioversion can do no good in the presence of asystole. It is worthwhile turning on the pacemaker in the hope that it may capture, but always remember that the mere presence of a pacing artefact does not necessarily mean that the heart is contracting. The third nurse should prepare the defibrillator and have the drugs ready. She or a fourth nurse will record and time all steps taken and all drugs given.

4   *Drugs needed:*

a   *Adrenaline solution,* 0·1 mg per ml (1 in 10 000 solution). Dose 1 to 2 ml intravenously (reaching the heart by cardiac massage), or by intracardiac injection, and repeated as necessary. A needle at least 4 in (10 cm) long should thus be at hand.

b   *Sodium bicarbonate solution,* 1·0 molar (1·0 mmol per ml). Dose 100 ml (100 mmol) by rapid infusion, repeated as necessary. Counteracting the metabolic acidosis present may be crucial to restoring a satisfactory rhythm.

c   *Calcium chloride solution,* 100 mg per ml (10 per cent solution). Dose 2 to 3 ml intravenously or into the heart.

d   *Lignocaine solution,* 20 mg per ml (2 per cent solution). Dose 1 to 2 mg per kg body weight, followed by a continuous infusion of 1 to 3 mg per min. The infusion can be made up in a paediatric drip set, 100 ml at a time; e.g. 15 ml of 2 per cent lignocaine plus 85 ml of 5 per cent glucose solution gives a concentration of 3 mg per ml. Lignocaine is of value only when cardiac arrest is due to ventricular fibrillation or tachycardia.

e   *Propranolol,* 1 mg per min for 5 min, may make the fibrillating ventricles more responsive to cardioversion. Sometimes marked hypotension may occur with a small dose of propranolol, which is only given when other measures have failed to restore a satisfactory rhythm.

f   *Isoprenaline* by continuous infusion of 0·1 to 1·0 μg per kg per min. A mixture of 0·2 mg (1 ampoule) in 100 ml of 5 per cent glucose solution gives a concentration of 2μg per ml. A constant-infusion pump should be used if one is available. Having restored a satisfactory rhythm it is essential to maintain cardiac output as close to normal levels as possible to minimise the risk of a further arrest.

g   *Dexamethasone* 8 mg, given intravenously, appears to reduce the effects of cerebral oedema. Dexamethasone acts more quickly than hydrocortisone.

5 Tracheal intubation, if not already done, will usually be necessary to ventilate the patient more effectively and to prevent the inhalation of vomit. A man usually needs a 9 mm tube, a woman an 8 mm tube and in infant a 3 or 4 mm uncuffed tube.
6 Relatives and (if appropriate) a clergyman must be informed.
7 Laboratory measurements of pH, blood gases and electrolyte levels are usually necessary. An arterial catheter ensures quick sampling of blood at a moment's notice, and should be put in if there is time; an arterial catheterization pack should thus be at hand.

Pulmonary embolism

After all operations, during confinement to bed, and in cardiac failure the formation of clots in the veins of the legs and pelvis is very common. Clots may form in the right atrium in atrial fibrillation. Should such a clot break away as an embolus it is carried to the lungs and lodges in a pulmonary artery. The result depends mainly on the size of the embolus. A big one obstructs a main pulmonary artery, causing shock and even sudden death. A medium-sized embolus blocks a smaller pulmonary artery, causing a *pulmonary infarct,* with dyspnoea, pleuritic pain, tachycardia, haemoptysis and fever. Myodardial infarction (p. 221) and spontaneous pneumothorax (p. 265) can mimic pulmonary embolism closely, and must be carefully excluded.

Prevention. Patients should not be confined to bed without good reason; but if they have to be, regular active or at least passive exercises diminish the risk of venous thrombosis. In cardiac failure and in atrial fibrillation the risk is high enough to warrant, at times, the prophylactic administration of an anticoagulant drug.

Treatment

1 Morphine is given for pain.
2 Oxygen in high concentration is needed when shock is present.
3 Digoxin and isoprenaline may be indicated when cardiac output is low.
4 An anticoagulant is given; it largely prevents further thrombosis and greatly reduces the chance of a second embolism. Heparin should be given at once and for several days followed by warfarin for a longer period (p. 236).

5 Removal of a big pulmonary embolus by means of bypass surgery may be possible and necessary. It will be preceded by a lung scan or pulmonary angiography if the patient's condition permits.

Myocardial infarction

Postoperatively this may occur (a) in older patients, (b) after operative cannulation of the coronary arteries, (c) after air embolism during operation; the last is usually presumptive. The features and treatment of myocardial infarction are described on p. 221. After operation its onset may be undramatic and a state of low cardiac output may be the only clue. Routine recording of all ECG leads and measurement of SGOT levels usually allow a diagnosis of myocardial infarction.

Renal failure

Postoperative renal complications are common. Renal function is impaired at this time by (a) a low cardiac output, renal blood flow and glomerular filtration rate (p. 96), (b) electrolyte disturbances and (c) tubular damage due to hypotension. Recovery is always possible except from renal infarction or cortical necrosis (p. 192).

   In practice, postoperative renal failure presents as oliguria (p. 96), and this must be managed in a methodical way.

Management of oliguria

1 Ensure that a low urinary flow is not due to retention of urine in the bladder. A catheter must usually be passed to find out.
2 Measure urinary output every 30 min. Collect in 12-hr lots and send each lot for estimation of creatinine, sodium and potassium content.
3 Blood urea and serum creatinine, sodium and potassium must be estimated every 12 hr.
4 Ensure that oliguria is not due to a low cardiac output (p. 190). Make sure that volume replacement is adequate; give volume expanders to achieve optimal filling pressures.
5 Ensure that oliguria is not due to dehydration. Restriction of water and sodium may have been too severe or, if a lot of blood has been given, the sodium and water needs may not have been met for

several hours. If urine osmolality is greater than 400 a response to fluid loading is likely. Test with a load of 300 ml of 5 per cent dextrose and, if a diuresis occurs, continue with relatively generous fluid replacement. In established renal failure urine osmolality is about 300.

6 Whatever the cause of the oliguria, urine flow may sometimes be restored by one or two large intravenous doses of frusemide, about 250 mg.

7 If there is no response to these measures, subsequent management is based on maintenance of fluid balance, hoping that recovery of renal function will occur. The regimen for anuria is designed to prevent urinary infection, to avoid digitalis poisoning, to replace water lost in the sweat, the breath and the urine, and to keep serum potassium concentration at a safe level.

a Urine collection and measurement, and blood tests, are continued.

b 'Barrier nursing' is started and suitable antibiotic drug(s) given. Aminoglycosides are stopped because failure to excrete them makes toxic damage almost certain.

c The dose of digoxin is reduced (p. 110).

d Water is given as 10 to 20 per cent glucose by infusion into the inferior vena cava, the total volume over 24 hr being 600 ml for 'insensible loss' plus the volume of the previous 24-hr urinary output. To this is added enough sodium chloride to replace the previous 24-hr urinary loss of sodium. In a hot environment insensible loss exceeds 600 ml.

e Serum potassium must not be allowed to exceed 7 mmol per l. Resonium A, 15 g 2 to 4 times per day orally or rectally, acts by binding potassium in the gut and thus preventing its reabsorption. Insulin, 10 to 20 units, 'covered' by 2 g of glucose per unit, acts by transporting potassium from the extracellular to the intracellular fluid.

Peritoneal dialysis is necessary if the measures under **e** fail to control serum K^+, and sometimes if blood urea grossly increases. For this procedure a fine plastic catheter with multiple small side holes is inserted into the abdominal cavity using either a trocar and cannula or a stilette placed down the inside of the catheter. The usual entry site is in the midline 2 centimetres below the umbilicus but, if this is not suitable, the lateral areas of the lower abdomen are used.

Through the catheter, dialysate fluid warmed to 37°C is run into the abdomen where it is left to equilibrate with the plasma circulating through the capillaries of the peritoneal membrane. The composition of dialysate fluid is such that sodium, chloride, calcium and magnesium are in concentrations equivalent to that in normal plasma; for convenience bicarbonate is replaced by an equivalent amount of lactate.

The principle of the technique is that the blood circulating through the capillaries in the peritoneal membrane is separated from the dialysate fluid by only the thin endothelial lining of the capillary and the slightly thicker peritoneal membrane. Water and small molecules pass through this membrane freely and move down concentration gradients. Thus, molecules such as urea and creatinine which are present in high concentration in the plasma and not present at all in the dialysate fluid, will move across the membrane and enter the peritoneal space. Equilibrium for these molecules is virtually complete in 30 to 35 minutes. Water will also move down concentration gradients and, to ensure that roughly equal amounts of fluid can be recovered from the peritoneum as was placed in it, glucose is added to the fluid to make it slightly hypertonic. The standard stock dialysate solution contains glucose at a concentration of 1·5 g per 100 ml. This has been found in the majority of patients to result in virtually equal amounts of fluid being returned as run in. On occasions, however, when it is required to remove more fluid than this, as for example when a patient has fluid overload and/or heart failure, the dialysate solution can be made even more hypertonic. Another stock dialysate solution has a glucose concentration of 7 g per 100 ml, and an intermediate concentration can be created by using mixtures of the two stock solutions.

The other variable content of peritoneal dialysis fluid is potassium. In most situations where peritoneal dialysis is being used, one of the indications is a high potassium level in the patient and usually the dialysate does not contain any potassium. However, this is not always appropriate and a stock solution containing 4 mmol per l potassium is available. Once again, an intermediate range of 2 mmol is easily obtainable by using equal volumes of the two stock solutions.

Fluid is usually run in by gravity in about ten minutes, left to equilibrate for 30 to 45 min, and then allowed to drain out by gravity into a separate container. The drainage procedure usually takes about 20 min. The cycle is then repeated. The volume of fluid used in an average adult is 2 litres. This amount may be reduced for small people or if the raised intra-abdominal pressure leads to respiratory embarrassment. The cycles are usually repeated continuously for about 36 hr and the catheter is then removed. Over this period of time the serum urea and creatinine levels could be expected to be roughly halved. The procedure can be restarted by replacing the catheter when required. The major problems relating to the technique are difficulties with drainage of fluid and infection. Meticulous technique is necessary, using great care to avoid introducing infection when the dialysis bottles are changed. In some units prophylactic antibiotics are added to the dialysis fluid to lessen this hazard.

Peritoneal dialysis is slower than haemodialysis but is more easily used in the ICU.

The recovery period. During recovery from acute tubular necrosis polyuria usually occurs, and loss of water, sodium and potassium during this phase is sometimes gross. The urinary losses have to be measured carefully and replaced until normal function returns.

Jaundice

Prolonged cardiac failure congests and scars the liver, and the extra metabolic load of an operation, coupled with the reduced hepatic blood flow which accompanies low cardiac output, may precipitate jaundice in such a patient. The problem may be accentuated in patients with a history of alcoholism or in patients with multivalve disease. With prolonged jaundice the possibility of hepatitis must be considered, although this is quite rare now with routine screening for hepatitis B antigen. The severity of liver damage can be gauged by the level of the serum bilirubin and of transaminase enzymes, AspAT and SGPT.

Jaundice is due to failure of bilirubin excretion. Encephalopathy may develop as the liver is unable to remove certain amino acids and ammonia derived from bacterial breakdown of protein in the bowel. Liver glycogen stores become depleted and hypoglycaemia may occur. The patient may show only minor confusion and agitation, or in the more advanced stages confusion may become marked and associated with a flapping tremor, deep coma may develop and eventually respiratory and circulatory disturbances may occur. Drug metabolism is impaired and sedatives must be used with great caution. An abnormal bleeding tendency develops because of impaired synthesis of clotting factors, often combined with abnormal platelet function. Ascites and oedema may develop because of failure of the liver to synthesize albumin.

Recovery is usual if further hepatic damage can be minimised. Hypoglycaemia is avoided by glucose infusion. The maximum concentration which can be given through a peripheral vein is 10 per cent but a concentration of up to 50 per cent may occasionally be required, given into a central vein. Vitamins, especially thiamine, are given as well, and vitamin K supplements ensure the maintenance of prothrombin if the liver is still able to make it. Sterilization of the bowel contents by oral neomycin (2 to 8 g daily) diminishes the absorption of toxins.

Diabetic ketoacidosis

With the increasing incidence of coronary arterial surgery in middle aged patients, management of diabetes has played an increasing role. Whatever the previous management, insulin therapy may well be required over the postoperative period. The underlying biochemical abnormality in diabetes is an absolute or relative deficiency of insulin. Glucose is not utilised by the tissues, hyperglycaemia develops and glucose escapes into the urine. Glycosuria causes an osmotic diuresis with large losses of water, sodium, chloride and potassium. In an attempt to overcome the problem of impaired glucose utilisation, the body breaks down adipose tissue. Excessive breakdown of fats leads to an accumulation of ketoacids in the blood with consequent metabolic acidosis. Because of the high sugar load given during cardiopulmonary bypass, hyperglycaemia is common anyway in the first postoperative hours and the stress of operation may temporarily overwhelm the body's homeostatic mechanisms. The usual signs of diabetic coma — thirst, polyuria, Kussmaul breathing, and altered state of consciousness — may, of course, be masked in this period so that constant vigilance is required.

Treatment consists of the administration of insulin, intravenous fluids and potassium. Treatment must be individualized according to the severity of the diabetes and the fluid and electrolyte balance of the patient. A common regimen would be administration of 10 units of soluble insulin per hr, reducing this to 5 units when blood sugar falls below 15 mmol per l and later according to urine test. Normal saline is given initially at a rate of 500 ml per hr for the first 2 to 3 hr, and then at a slower rate, reverting to dextrose-saline when blood sugar is controlled. Much less sodium chloride is commonly required in postoperative patients. Remember that signs of hypoglycaemia, especially sweating and tachycardia, may be masked by beta blocking drugs.

Cerebral complications

These may present as:
1 *Weakness or paralysis,* commonly of hemiplegic distribution, due to thrombosis (especially in older patients) or embolism (by a clot from a fibrillating atrium or inserted prosthetic mitral or aortic valve) of a cerebral artery.
2 *Convulsions,* which may be focal (face or limb) or generalized. Convulsions often denote diffuse cerebral oedema, which may follow prolonged hypotension with a reduction in cerebral blood flow, or cerebral embolism. Unexplained fitting without hemiparesis may result from air embolism with a diffuse distribution. Fits may also be due to a hypocalcaemia or hypoglycaemia.

Prevention. Clot embolism, often a late event, may be forestalled by long-term anticoagulant treatment in patients at special risk (see p. 236).

Treatment

A fit, however minor, requires immediate investigation and treatment:
a Diazepam, up to 20 mg by slow intravenous injection, is usually the best immediate treatment.
b Phenobarbitone, 100 to 200 mg 8 or 12-hourly provides more prolonged protection. Sometimes phenytoin, up to 4 mg per kg intravenously over 5 min followed by 100 mg 6-hourly, may be added. Where oral treatment is possible the preferred treatment is to give an initial loading dose of 1·0 g of phenytoin.

c   If minor fits break through despite the above measures, paral-
dyhyde 5 to 10 ml IV may be given intermittently.

d   Repeated convulsions so interfere with ventilation that artificial
ventilation must usually be started; repeated anoxia is a dangerous
insult in the early postoperative period.

e   Paralysis with tubocurarine may be necessary if convulsions
cannot be adequately controlled. This is rare.

f   Steroid, e.g. dexamethasone 8 mg intramuscularly followed by 4
mg every 6 hr, helps reduce cerebral oedema. Cerebral oedema is
an inevitable accompaniment of fitting and can in itself worsen the
situation.

g   Mannitol (p. 108) does not enter cells and by osmotic action
attracts water from the cells into the extracellular compartment; it is
useful in the emergency treatment of convulsions. Administration
of a diuretic, usually frusemide, may also play a role.

3   *Prolonged coma.* Although the rate of recovery from anaesthesia varies, especially in critically ill patients who have had a long
operation, concern arises about the possibility of cerebral damage
in the patient who is slow to wake. Assessment of the progress of a
patient in prolonged coma requires a systematic approach. The
following summary is based on the Glasgow Coma Scale.

a   *Eye opening:* Spontaneous and purposeful; in response to
speech; in response to pain; none.

b   *Verbal response:* Oriented; confused and disorientated; inap-
propriate (e.g. calling out at random); incomprehensible (-
meaningless moaning); none.

c   *Motor response:* obeys commands; responds to pain (pencil on a
nail bed, squeezed upper fibres of trapezius muscle or squeezed
achilles tendon); (1) Localised (affected limb); (2) extensor posturing (Fig. 60), (a) decorticate rigidity indicating damage of the
corticospinal tracts in the cerebral hemispheres. It may also be
provoked by tracheal suctioning (b) decerebrate rigidity indicating
damage to the cerebral hemispheres and the upper brain stem (the
midbrain and pons); (3) none.

Sudden deterioration of the state of consciousness may indicate
coning, i.e. herniation of brain structures through the tentorium and
foramen magnum due to cerebral oedema. Specific signs of this
event are:

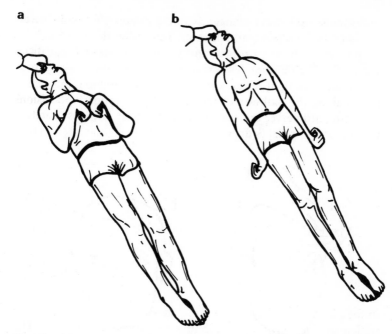

Fig. 60 (a) Decorticate rigidity; flexion of the arms, wrists and fingers, with extension of the legs (see text) and (b) decerebrate rigidity; arching of the back and extension of the arms and legs, sometimes accompanied by overbreathing.

a Deterioration in level of consciousness.
b Dilatation of pupil and loss of pupillary light reflex on one or both sides.
c Increased tone.
d Respiratory dysfunction, arterial hypertension and bradycardia. Urgent treatment of cerebral oedema is required with steroid, mannitol, diuretics and hyperventilation. Lowering the P_{CO_2} to 3·3 kPa (25 mmHg) constricts cerebral vessels and lowers intracranial pressure.

Pupillary responses. The pupil dilates with sympathetic stimulus and constricts with parasympathetic stimulus, the latter passing from the midbrain with the 3rd nerve. Cerebral anoxia dilates both pupils and persistence of dilatation beyond a few minutes usually indicates severe brain damage. Coning dilates the pupils and a lesion in the pons (sympathetic centre) constricts them. It must also be remembered that atropine and sympathomimetic drugs dilate the pupils and that opiates constrict them.

An impaired light reflex, with a fixed, dilated pupil, indicates a lesion along the pathway of the reflex arc — retina, optic nerve, midbrain, 3rd nerve; in a comatosed patient the lesion is usually in the midbrain or the 3rd nerve.

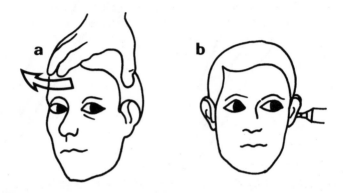

Fig. 61 (a) The normal doll's eye response. The head is rotated sharply to the right; the eyes move to the left and (b) the normal caloric reflex. Twenty ml of ice cold water are syringed into the left ear; the eyes turn to the left. Reflexes are tested on both sides.

Eye movements further assist in localizing a cerebral lesion. A normal corneal reflex (blink + upward eye movement) indicates brain stem function between the 5th nerve nucleus (afferent) and 3rd nerve nucleus (efferent). A normal doll's-eye response (Fig. 61a) and caloric reflex (Fig. 61b) show normal function between the 8th nerve (afferent) and the nerves supplying the eye muscles (3rd, 4th and 6th).

Prognosis in coma. Many patients will recover fully from profound coma but it is rare for this to happen when there are no signs of improvement after 1 or 2 weeks. Clearly life support must be maintained while there is any chance of survival with recovery but, equally clearly, it is undesirable from all points of view to continue ventilatory and other support when severe, irreversible brain damage is present. Signs indicating this are:

a Profound coma.

b Absent brain stem reflexes, i.e. fixed pupils, absent corneal, doll's-eye and caloric reflexes, absent cough and gag reflex, absence of spontaneous respiration.

Depression of responses by drugs or hypothermia must be excluded and arterial PCO_2 must be normal when respiratory activity is tested. It is important to appreciate that purely spinal reflexes, such as flexion on response to painful stimuli, may persist even in the presence of gross brain damage.

An EEG may be recorded but it is not essential. Before withdrawing support, however, it is mandatory to have a specialist neurological opinion. It is also mandatory that relatives shall be fully informed and prepared for withdrawal of support. It may sometimes be necessary to continue treatment for an extra period before this difficult adjustment can be made.

Psychiatric complications

To be a patient in an ICU is an unenviable experience and it is not surprising that psychological upsets occur. These are revealed as withdrawal from reality, overdependence, confusion, depression, aggression, delusions and hallucinations. Physical causes of mental symptoms must be carefully sought; these include:

1 Water depletion or intoxication, sodium or potassium depletion (p. 13).

2 Hypoxia, hypercapnia; sometimes hypocapnia.

3 Acidosis, alkalosis.

4 Pain, urinary retention, faecal impaction, inability to communicate.

5 Cerebral complications.

A toxic confusional state may exist because of the trauma of postoperative experience, fever and multiple minor biochemical anomalies, all in a foreign and rather threatening environment. The emphasis in management is improvement of the physical state and nutrition as rapidly as possible, rest and privacy, minimising disturbance and discomfort, and allowing family to be present as much as possible. Temporary sedation may be required and psychiatric advice should be sought for a major disturbance.

Chapter 9

Respiratory problems

Maintenance of adequate ventilation is vital in the postoperative period and is discussed in detail on pages 241–262.

Special problems in particular conditions

1 *Atrial fibrillation* and *prosthetic valves* are prone to cause embolism and justify long-term anticoagulant treatment. Homograft valves do not. If, however, the homograft is mounted on a support or 'stent', emboli may arise from the stent in the early postoperative period. An anticoagulant is thus commonly given to these patients and to patients with other stent mounted bioprostheses for 3 to 6 weeks after operation.

2 After resection of an aortic *coarctation,* hypertension is common in the first few days and may have to be controlled with vasodilator drugs (p. 118). Mesenteric arteritis rarely occurs, leading to ileus or even infarction of the gut. Hypertension may also require control in other conditions, particularly after valve replacement.

3 When mitral disease, ventricular septal defect, patent ductus or any other condition is accompanied by a *high pulmonary vascular resistance,* surgery may precipitate severe right heart failure. The resistance is controlled as far as possible by maintenance of optimal blood gases, with control both of respiration and cardiac output. The vasodilating action of isoprenaline is useful and occasionally other vasodilators are required. Almost all vasodilators affect the pulmonary vascular resistance similarly to the systemic vascular resistance.

4 *Persistent pyrexia* usually results from haematoma or infection of the wound, respiratory or urinary tracts; sometimes a postpericardotomy or postbypass syndrome may develop within a week of operation. For any persistent pyrexia, however, blood cultures are required to exclude the possibility of bacterial or fungal endocarditis. Fortunately such complications are rare but further surgery is required on occasion. When shock and fever occur together, septicaemia is often due to a *Gram-negative organism;* these infections are a special danger after catheterization of the bladder.

Death in the intensive care unit

Inevitably death in the ICU is an only too frequent event. When staff have expended all energy in the care of the living, support of the bereaved can receive inadequate attention. All staff have a clear understanding of their responsibilities and competence in the care of the living. Once death occurs, responsibilities are less clear and some feel uncertain about their competence to cope with the situation. The problem is compounded by personal disappointment at the outcome, and a feeling of responsibility for the failure of medical treatment. Yet in some ways the support of relatives after the death of a patient is one of the most important tasks in the ICU, requiring a sympathetic and skilled approach from all staff.

Although no one can completely answer the immediate question 'why did this happen?' families turn for explanation to those professionals they see as competent and knowledgeable. Medical and nursing staff can give medical explanations, a necessary first step if the family is to grieve appropriately. Assisting relatives through the first difficult moments and liaising with other staff such as social workers and chaplains are important roles for nurses and are of great value to the patient's family. Relatives have passed through a period of great tension, ending in the disaster they had always feared. First emotions are an overwhelming mixture of grief, disbelief and a bleak, exhausted emptiness. The ICU has become an unpleasant place and yet it is the last place of contact with the patient. Staff often fear they will intrude on a private grief, but this is seldom how relatives see their presence. They are bewildered and distraught, and caring, practical assistance is seen as helpful, rather than as an intrusion. More often the family feels rejected if staff are not nearby; rejected first by the patient's loss of life, second by the fact that staff seem involved with others.

The provision of a quiet room, a telephone call to friends, an explanation of what the hospital or the law requires, and of who to contact, are all supportive. The family will want to know at a relatively early stage whether a postmortem examination is required, although they might not wish to make an immediate decision if the choice is theirs. These steps bridge the first period and allow time for family members to recover their strength and marshall their resources.

The question of what to say is best solved by sensitive listening. You can do little more; your presence is what is needed, and then possibly a referral to another staff member. Those families with church affiliation will ask for the chaplain or priest, others may value his presence but not think to ask. A social worker may already have a relationship with the patient's family, and can usefully support them through this stressful time, facilitating their departure from the hospital and reinforcing the family's own capacity to deal with the death. Some of the needs of families from a different culture can be easily overlooked; special care should be taken to recognize and help meet these needs.

Dealing with death in the ICU is a difficult task for all staff. Carried out perfunctorily and without sensitivity it can add emotional scars which never heal; carried out caringly and sensitively it is of inestimable value to the bereaved family. Detailed discussion is beyond the scope of this book, but further reading from appropriate texts is recommended.

10   Ischaemic Heart Disease

Atherosclerosis is now the main cause of death in affluent countries. It is characterized by the deposition of fatty substances in the walls of arteries varying in size from the aorta to the coronary arteries. These deposits take the form of small knobs or plaques; they may narrow the lumen or fill it in small arteries, or they may ulcerate through the arterial lining and favour thrombosis on the roughened area so formed.

When an artery is narrowed, the tissues it supplies are inadequately supplied with blood, a state termed *ischaemia*. If the narrowing is gradual, an alternative blood supply may develop by the enlargement of smaller arteries which bypass the obstruction; this is the *collateral circulation* to the area. Should the main artery be narrowed or blocked before the collateral circulation has time to develop, the tissue it supplies dies; the necrotic region is then termed an *infarct* except in the case of a limb which is described as *gangrenous*.

The involvement of coronary arteries in atherosclerosis is very common, and its consequences are especially serious in so vital an organ as the heart. The condition is known by the general term *ischaemic heart disease*, which manifests itself by angina of effort, myocardial infarction or sudden death. The cause of ischaemic heart disease, or of atherosclerosis in general is unknown, but several predisposing causes have been recognized:

1 *Heredity.* The disease tends to run in families.
2 *Hypertension.*
3 *Hyperlipidaemia*, the most common factor being raised serum cholesterol. The damaging cholesterol appears to be that carried in low density lipoproteins; high density lipoprotein cholesterol appears protective.
4 *Cigarette smoking.*

217

These are the four main risk factors. Obesity is also unfavourable, perhaps mainly because of its association with hypertension and hyperlipidaemia. Diabetes and gout are also unfavourable, as are lack of exercise and emotional stress. To a degree atherosclerosis is inevitable with increasing age, but factors in the Western way of life have greatly accelerated the process.

The natural history of coronary arterial disease

Significant atheromatous narrowings of the coronary arteries may be present for 20 years or more without symptoms. Development of complications from a given lesion depends on the site and severity of the lesion and on the extent of disease in other vessels.

Anginal pain occurs when cardiac muscle is inadequately supplied with oxygen. Lactic acid, produced by anaerobic metabolism (p. 21) in the ischaemic area, stimulates nerve endings to produce a characteristic pain. Angina is usually related to effort, but may occur at rest and sometimes is no more than a minor tightness in the chest, readily eased by rest or sublingual nitroglycerine. In more severe bouts the pain is crushing or constricting, felt in the front of the chest, either centrally or right across; it may spread into the neck, lower jaw and arms. It may be hard to distinguish from the pain of massive pulmonary embolism, pericarditis, oesophagitis and dissecting aneurysm of the aorta. Correlation with coronary arteriography has shown that atypical pain may be associated with severe coronary arterial disease. An ECG during pain or exercise has proved valuable in distinguishing the subgroup at high risk of further complications. Marked ST depression or elevation, frequent ventricular premature beats or a drop in blood pressure are ominous features requiring further investigation.

When anginal-type pain continues for longer than 20 min or so the attack is often described as a bout of *myocardial ischaemia.* Angina may progress to *myocardial infarction*, or a patient may develop a malignant arrhythmia; indeed sudden ventricular fibrillation may be the first sign of coronary artery disease (Fig. 62).

Given that severe underlying coronary arterial disease is usually present, it is not always clear what triggers myocardial infarction. *Thrombosis* may occur on an atheromatous plaque or *haemorrhage* within it; either event may occlude a coronary artery or critically narrow it so that muscle supplied by the vessel is non-viable. A

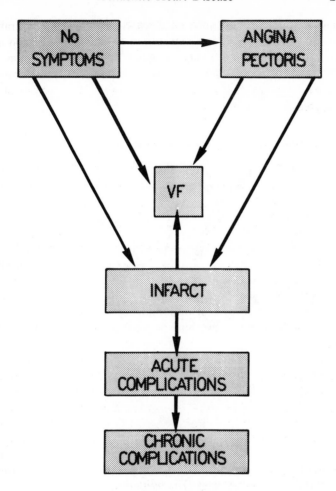

Fig. 62 The natural history of coronary arterial disease. Patients may return to having no symptoms, or having angina pectoris, at any stage.

plaque may rupture, occluding smaller distal vessels by embolism of its contents. It is now clear, however, that these events occur with only a minority of infarcts. Spasm of the artery or formation of platelet aggregates with peripheral embolism may trigger some; both processes are known to occur and can, on occasion, cause angina or trigger an infarct even in the absence of severe atheromatous coronary arterial disease. Alternatively a sudden demand on the circulation may prove too much for an area of myocardium which has a very marginal blood supply.

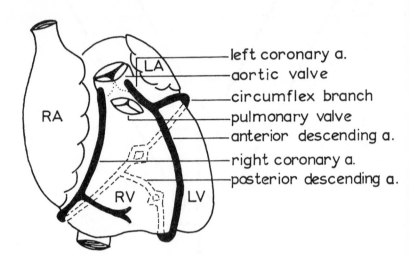

Fig. 63 Anatomy of the coronary arteries. RA, right atrium; LA, left atrium; RV, right ventricle; LV, left ventricle.

Anatomy of the coronary arteries (Fig. 63)

The right and left coronary arteries arise from the aorta just above two of the aortic valve cusps. The *right* one winds round the groove between atria and ventricles, supplying branches to the right ventricle and right atrium. Behind the heart it supplies a branch to the atrioventricular (A-V) node. Finally it gives off the *posterior descending artery* and then anastomoses with the end of the circumflex artery. The posterior descending artery passes from the A-V groove to the apex of the heart, supplying adjacent areas of the left and right ventricles as it goes.

The *left* coronary artery soon divides into a circumflex branch, which winds to the left and backwards along the A-V groove to join the right coronary artery, supplying the left atrium and ventricle as it goes, and the *anterior descending branch*. The latter passes from the A-V groove to the apex of the heart, supplying adjacent areas of the left and right ventricles on the way. The interventricular septum is supplied, in front, by the anterior descending artery and, behind by the posterior descending artery.

Myocardial infarction is mainly a disease of the left ventricle although infarction of the right ventricle may be quite extensive in inferior infarction due to occlusion of the right coronary artery. Narrowing of the right coronary artery affects the posterior and inferior parts of the left ventricle, and may cause A-V block (p. 161) because this vessel supplies the A-V node. Narrowing of the anterior descending artery affects the anterior and septal ('anteroseptal') regions and may cause left or right bundle branch block, or both when infarction is extensive. Narrowing of the circumflex artery affects the anterolateral part of the left ventricle and its postero-inferior surface.

Myocardial infarction

Typically, the patient (who may or may not previously have had angina) is struck with anginal pain lasting from 30 min to several hours, is seen to be cold, sweating, pale and anxious. The heart rate is variable, but bradycardia (due to vagal overactivity) is more common than tachycardia at the onset of infarction. The blood

a   **b**   **c**

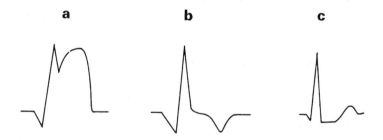

Fig. 64 ECG changes in myocardial infarction and acute coronary insufficiency. (a) Acute myocardial infarction. The ST segment is elevated with an upward convexity. The broad, deep Q wave indicates full-thickness infarction. (b) Late myocardial infarction. The Q wave persists, the ST segment has returned to normal and the T wave is inverted. (c) Acute coronary insufficiency. The ST segment is depressed. Diagrammatic.

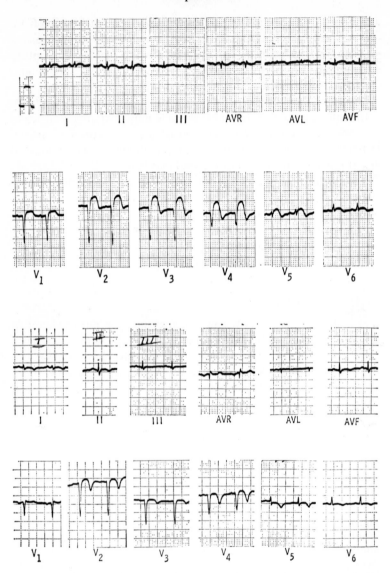

Fig. 65 Anterior myocardial infarction (*top*) 10 hours from the onset of infarction. The changes of acute infarction are seen in the precordial leads V₂ to V₆ (*bottom*). Tracing from the same patient one month later. The changes of late infarction are now seen in the precordial leads. Both ECGs show less marked changes in the postero-interior leads, II, III and AVF.

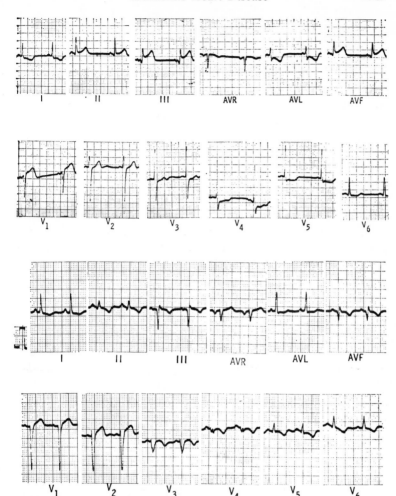

Fig. 66 Postero-inferior myocardial infarction. (*top*) 12 hr from the onset of infarction. The changes of acute infarction are shown in the postero-inferior leads, 2, 3 and AVF. (*bottom*) Tracing from the same patient 5 weeks later. The changes of late infarction are now seen in the postero-inferior leads. Less marked changes in precordial leads indicate some extension to the anterior surface of the heart. At 12 hr ST depression was evident in the anterolateral leads. This is often seen opposite an infarct and is referred to as *reciprocal ST depression*. The tracing at 5 weeks, however, shows that, at some stage, infarction has extended well around on to the anterior surface.

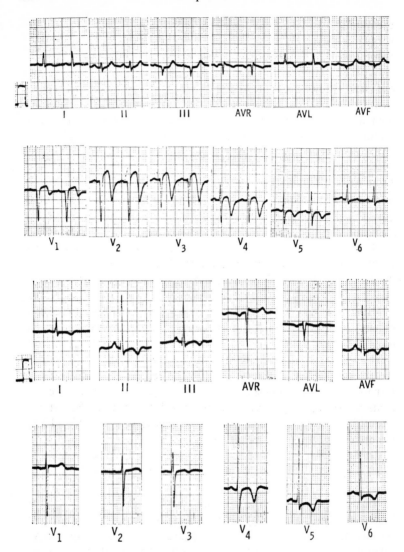

Fig. 67 (*top*) Antero-septal infarction, 8 days from the onset of infarction. ST segments are returning to normal and the T waves are inverted. Changes are most marked in leads V₁ to V₄. (*bottom*) Antero-lateral infarction, 3 weeks after onset. The ST segments are normal and the T waves are inverted. Changes are most marked in leads V₄ to V₆ but there is some extension to the postero-inferior leads II, III and AVF. The absence of abnormal Q waves shows that the infarct was subendocardial.

pressure is frequently high due to sympathetic overactivity. With a very large infarct the heart rate is rapid and the blood pressure low. Sometimes pain is atypical and dyspnoea or profound weakness may predominate; in a few cases infarction may be genuinely 'silent', being diagnosed later when the patient has a routine electrocardiogram or dies and has a postmortem examination. There is a high incidence of ventricular fibrillation, often fatal, in the first minutes or hours of an attack.

The diagnosis is confirmed by electrocardiography and enzyme studies. The ECG (Fig. 64–67) shows the following changes:

1 If the infarct involves the whole thickness of the ventricular wall, a *Q wave* will be prominent over the infarct. Some infarcts involve only the deeper layers (subendocardial) and do not produce an abnormal Q wave. The distinction between subendocardial and full thickness infarcts is only an approximation but, in general, the greater the muscle loss the greater the loss of R wave.

2 The *ST interval* (or segment) is raised above the baseline in the early stages. During the next 2 to 10 days the ST segment falls to the baseline and the T wave becomes inverted. When ST elevation persists longer than this, the presence of a ventricular aneurysm must be suspected.

These changes appear in different leads according to the site of the infarct. A posteroinferior infarct (posterior descending artery territory) shows itself in leads 2, 3 and AVF; anteroseptal infarction (anterior descending territory) shows in V1, V2 and V3; anterolateral infarcts (circumflex territory) affect leads V4, V5 and V6. Combined patterns may be seen.

Confirmatory evidence may be sought from *changes in the blood.* The leucocyte count rises above 10 000 per mm^3 and the sedimentation rate above 10 mm in 1 hr. More importantly, enzymes in the serum, e.g. glutamic-aspartate aminotranferase (AspAT), creatine kinase (CK) and α hydroxybutyric dehydrogenase (HBD), increase because they are released from dead cardiac muscle (AspAt above 50 units per l, CK above 190 units per l, HBD above 200 units per l). Enzyme changes occur in other diseases; for instance CK is raised in muscle necrosis, AspAT in hepatic disease and HBD in haemolytic anaemia. Measurement of CKMB, the isoenzyme of CK released from the heart, is therefore preferred in some units. Measurement of CKMB is rather laborious and a battery of the three other tests (which can be automated) gives similar information. CK is usually raised from 12 to 48 hr, AspAT from 1 to 4 days and HBD from 2 to 7 days, after infarction. The diagnosis of myocardial infarction can be considered secure if two of the three main features are present; these are typical and prolonged chest pain, typical ECG change, and typical enzyme change.

Complications

Arrhythmias are most likely to occur within the first 3 days, particularly within the first 24 hr, of infarction. Sinus bradycardia may occur in the first few hours. Ventricular fibrillation, the critical arrhythmia, is sometimes preceded by salvos of ventricular ectopic beats but sometimes occurs without prior warning. The development of complete heart block may be an ominous feature after anterior infarction. Atrial arrhythmias tend to occur later and are usually relatively easily managed.

2 *Left ventricular failure* may occur with an extensive infarct, producing tachypnoea, pulmonary venous congestion and signs of lowered cardiac output.

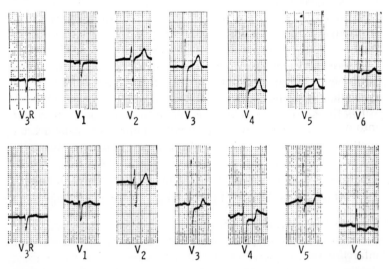

Fig. 68 Acute coronary insufficiency. (*top*) Tracing when pain was not present. (*bottom*) Tracing recorded during prolonged chest pain. ST segments are depressed in leads V₃ to V₆.

3 *Frank cardiogenic shock* may occur and carries a grave prognosis.

4 *Rupture of the ventricular wall* occasionally occurs at the site of a full thickness infarct, and is rapidly fatal. Rupture of an infarcted papillary muscle causes mitral regurgitation, and of the ventricular septum a ventricular septal defect; both these conditions may sometimes be repaired surgically.

5 *Systemic embolism* may occur from a thrombus on the endocardial surface of the infarct.

6 *Pulmonary embolism* may occur, particularly in an immobile patient with a low cardiac output.

7 The weakened ventricular wall at the site of the infarct may gradually give way with formation of an *aneurysm*. This may produce progressive left ventricular failure or it may be associated with bouts of ventricular tachycardia and ventricular fibrillation.

8 A *post-infarction syndrome* with fever, pericarditis and continued pain is an uncommon event, occurring from approximately one week after infarction.

Acute coronary insufficiency (Fig. 68)

This term is given to an attack which clinically is indistinguishable from myocardial infarction, but in which even prolonged anginal pain is not accompanied by ECG or enzyme confirmation of an infarct. The ECG usually shows *depression of the ST segment* below the baseline, for as long as the pain lasts. Sometimes there may be *fluctuating elevation of the ST segment* interspersed with intervals where the ECG is normal. Acute coronary insufficiency may turn into a frank infarct at any time; where marked ST changes are a feature, early coronary arteriography and operation are usually required.

Management of the patient with myocardial infarction

The mortality of patients presenting with a new, sudden coronary event, including those who collapse with an arrhythmia before frank infarction can occur, is 30 to 40 per cent. Over 60 per cent of these deaths occur before the patient can be brought to hospital. The outlook of a patient stricken with ventricular fibrillation will be determined in the next 2 or 3 min. Education of the public in basic cardiopulmonary resuscitation has therefore become part of the function of a coronary care unit (CCU). Life-Support Units have also developed in association with the CCU. A life-support ambulance is staffed by two paramedical personnel who, having assessed the situation (with the family doctor if present), attempt to stabilise the patient's condition to allow safe transport to the CCU. An ECG is obtained and, if necessary, transmitted by radio to the CCU for help in diagnosis. Sinus bradycardia is treated with atropine, ventricular fibrillation is treated with cardioversion, and cardiac massage is performed if required, usually ventilating by means of an oropharyngeal airway. Lignocaine is given if needed by intravenous infusion.

The patient is admitted directly to the CCU where constant professional observation, assessment and care is possible. The goals of management are:

1 The alleviation of symptoms, particularly pain, fear and anxiety.
2 The prevention or early detection and treatment of dangerous arrhythmias.
3 The prevention or treatment of cardiac failure and shock.
4 The prevention of embolism.
5 Rehabilitation and education of the patient and his family.

Initial procedures on admission

The patient's condition is assessed immediately on admission to the CCU. *Pain*, in addition to distressing the patient, further stresses the heart and increases the tendency to shock. It is commonly treated with morphine, usually 10 mg IV, or pentazocine 30 mg IV. *A low output state* is suggested by restlessness, dyspnoea, tachycardia or hypotension. Immediate treatment (p. 190) is required. Even if he is relatively comfortable, the patient will be apprehensive about his condition and uncertain about the fate awaiting him in the CCU. His condition should be explained to him, he should be reassured in a quiet but confident manner, and routine procedures should be explained briefly and simply to him. Remember that anxiety may alter the patient's perception and that he may not recall explanations.

Immediately after preliminary assessment preparations are made for ECG monitoring.

ECG monitoring. Skin electrodes are attached according to the instructions with the electrode sets, shaving the chest if necessary. MCL1 is usually the best lead (Fig. 51). Good contacts are ensured by cleaning the skin with alcohol and applying enough electrode paste, or by using pre-gelled electrodes. The electrode lead is plugged into the bedside oscilloscope which is wired to another oscilloscope in the central nursing station; this in turn connects with the direct-writing recorder. The monitor sweep is kept at 6 sec, the gain is set to give a QRS complex of about 2 cm, the position is set to keep the QRS in the middle of the screen and the alarm is turned off. Other settings vary with different monitoring systems and the routine for each unit can be readily mastered.

At the central station the alarm is set at the high and low positions, but in restless patients both may have to be set at 'low' or even

Coronary Care Chart

Early Progress Sheet

(Progress to be reported hourly or as directed)

Surname: SMITH | MR | 11 | 401 C2244

Christian names: JOHN HENRY | M | 28·1·25 | 56 | Auckland

Address: 20 South Road, GREENLANE. | Dom. Code | Clinical Team: DR GREEN

Date: 4·2·81 | C.C.No. 201

Time	Heart rate	Blood pressure	Chest pain	Arrhythmias: Sinus rhythm A F etc	Arrhythmias: Ectopics	Temperature	Respiration	Analgesic and antiarrhythmic drugs
1000	110	150/100	Mild	ST	occasional VPBs	37°C	26	Glyceryl trinitrate 0·6mg S.L.
1100	120	150/105 – 145/100	Nil	ST	Short run VT 6 beats, rate 190			1115 Lignocaine bolus 100mg Lignocaine infusion 3mg/min
1200	105	140/95	Nil	ST	isolated VPBs			Lignocaine infusion 3mg/min
1300	100	140/90	Nil	ST	nil seen			" " " "
1400	100		Nil	ST	" "	37·5 °C	22	" " " "
1500	95		Nil	SR	" "			Lignocaine infusion 2mg/min

Fig. 69 Record-sheet of a patient in the coronary care unit.

turned off. The recorder gain is set to give a QRS complex of about 2 cm and the stylus is centred so that both normal and ectopic complexes are recorded on the paper. Recordings are usually made at 25 mm per sec and in general are best made from the central station.

Some monitoring systems incorporate other features including:

1 An alarm to indicate that one of the electrodes has been dislodged, to avoid the erroneous conclusion that the patient has developed asystole.

2 A 'memory' tape loop so that electrical events leading to an arrhythmia can be recorded permanently. With this system the ECG pattern is recorded continuously on a magnetic tape. When an arrhythmia occurs the tracing of the previous 15 to 30 sec is printed out automatically.

3 An alarm or magnetic-tape printout can be triggered by ECG changes other than rate changes, for example by widening of the QRS with the development of bundle branch block or with ventricular ectopics.

Each of these systems has its advantages. For most patients a simple system of monitoring combined with vigilant nursing is all that is necessary.

On-going assessment. Progress and treatment are recorded in the coronary care record sheets. Assessment and recording routines vary with each Unit, but a typical chart is shown in Fig. 69 and an appropriate recording system is as follows: hourly recordings of the heart rate are made by counting from the central station monitor (not from the rate monitor which is often inaccurate) and the number of ectopic beats in 1 min are recorded similarly. A 10-second strip is recorded hourly on the direct writer and this strip is subsequently mounted. Ectopic beats or other arrhythmias occurring outside the routine recording period are of course noted and recorded if significant.

Blood pressure is recorded every 2 hr for 12 hr and then 4-hourly. If the systolic pressure falls below 100 mmHg, however, hourly recordings are made.

A 13-lead ECG is recorded on each of the first 2 to 3 days. The routine haematological and biochemical tests are made on the day of admission while serum AspAt, CK and HBD levels (or CKMB levels) are recorded daily on the first 3 to 4 days. Temperature is recorded 4-hourly.

Maintenance of physical comfort. The patient must be allowed to rest in a comfortable position as far as possible, as rest decreases the stress on the heart. Unless the patient is shocked he is nursed in a semi-upright position. This position is comfortable and minimises pulmonary venous congestion by reducing the pulmonary blood volume.

Attention to hygiene and pressure areas is essential, but the regimen should be flexible to permit as much rest as possible. Although the shocked patient must be kept at rest, those who are not distressed frequently find the use of a bedside commode less taxing than balancing on a bed pan. A brief period sitting in a chair is allowed from the first day in uncomplicated cases. A light, attractive and nutritious diet is offered.

Detection and treatment of arrhythmias

About 90 per cent of patients develop an arrhythmia after myocardial infarction. This may be dangerous, even when the infarct is small and the patient capable of full recovery. The chapter on arrhythmias should be revised in conjunction with this section. *Ventricular fibrillation* is the dangerous arrhythmia, but other arrhythmias are reviewed briefly.

Arrhythmias arising in the sinus node

Sinus tachycardia, with a persistent rate above 100 per min, signifies extensive myocardial damage and low cardiac output (p. 147). *Sinus bradycardia* is common in the first few hours and is usually due to a vagal reflex (p. 147). It does not usually require treatment but, where necessary, may be abolished by atropine (0·4 to 0·6 mg). *Sinus arrest* for a few seconds at a time is unusual but may herald cardiac standstill. *Sinus arrhythmia* and *wandering pacemaker* are unimportant.

Supraventricular arrhythmias

Supraventricular arrhythmias are not usually troublesome in the early stages of myocardial infarction. *Ectopic beats* may lead to supraventricular tachycardia (p. 152) or atrial fibrillation (p. 153). *Supreventricular tachycardia* and *atrial fibrillation* may reduce cardiac output and aggravate failure if they continue for some time, more frequently they subside spontaneously without treatment. After myocardial infarction digitalis is more than usually likely to cause dangerous ventricular arrhythmias, and should be used with caution. Cardioversion is, therefore, often preferred in the initial treatment of these arrhythmias (if treatment is needed), but digitalis is usually necessary when atrial fibrillation is persistent.

Ventricular arrhythmias

Ectopic beats are common. Occurring in salvos they often lead to ventricular tachycardia; when they coincide with the T wave of the preceding beat, ventricular fibrillation is likely to develop. They can be suppressed with lignocaine, if necessary with the addition of procainamide or other drugs (p. 155).

Ventricular tachycardia may seriously reduce cardiac output or produce pulmonary oedema. When this arrhythmia occurs in the first 24 hr after infarction, however, the arrhythmia is usually transient, lasting 10 seconds or less. Episodes of this arrhythmia occurring late, usually beyond 1 week, are more likely to be serious. If, at its onset, the patient becomes breathless or loses consciousness, cardioversion must be carried out at once; otherwise there is time to try other treatment (p. 157). Sometimes after myocardial infarction, but rarely otherwise, the QRS complex looks like that of ventricular tachycardia but the rate is less than 100 per min (Fig. 70). This commonly occurs in the presence of sinus bradycardia or sinus arrhythmia. This relatively slow arrhythmia is best termed

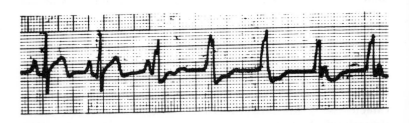

Fig. 70 Accelerated idioventricular rhythm.

'accelerated idioventricular rhythm'; it often reverts spontaneously to sinus rhythm and, provided haemodynamic status is satisfactory, it is not routinely treated. *Ventricular fibrillation* and *cardiac standstill* (asystole) are grave emergencies; their management is described on p. 201. Ventricular fibrillation may occur even when the infarct is relatively small and haemodynamic status appears satisfactory. Provided immediate cardioversion is carried out, further progress may be quite uneventful although type 1 anti-arrhythmic drugs (p. 111) are usually given to reduce the risk of further bouts.

Defects of conduction

Right bundle branch block may herald the occurrence of complete A-V block (p. 164). *Complete A-V block* is of variable significance; (a) with posteroinferior infarction the ventricular rate is often not very low and the block resolves without incident; (b) only a big anterior infarct produces A-V block; the rate is low, the patient shocked and death is common. In either case the appropriate treatment (p. 164) should be readily available, but intracardiac pacing is more often necessary in the case of anterior infarction in which A-V block is such a grave complication.

Treatment of LV failure and shock

With a sizeable myocardial infarction, cardiac output falls and left ventricular filling pressure rises. Provided stable conditions can be maintained and extension of the infarct does not occur, gradual improvement and uneventful recovery are possible. If the patient deteriorates into frank shock the outlook is grave, survival being about 20 per cent and death in subsequent months common in survivors. Optimal treatment of left ventricular failure is therefore required to try and avoid the perils of frank shock. Efforts have been made to improve the assessment of haemodynamic status and to tailor treatment precisely to the patient's needs. An estimate of left atrial, and hence left ventricular filling pressure, can be obtained from a wedged pulmonary arterial pressure. When a catheter is wedged peripherally in a pulmonary arterial branch, flow through that branch ceases; the pressure in left atrium and pulmonary veins is then transmitted through the capillary bed to the distal lumen of the catheter. This recording is made with a Swan-Ganz balloon catheter. If a thermodilution catheter is used, cardiac output can then be measured after the catheter is withdrawn to a free position in the pulmonary artery. Knowing cardiac index and left atrial pressure, treatment can be planned as in Fig. 71. With a satisfactory cardiac output and acceptable left atrial pressure (left upper quadrant), no treatment may be required. With a low filling pressure but low cardiac output (left lower quadrant), volume

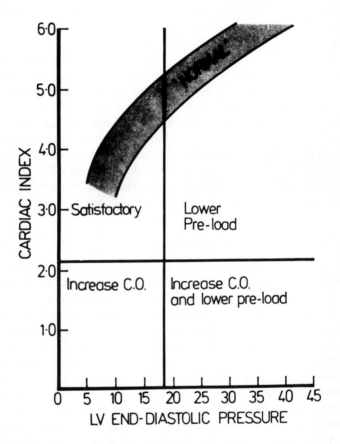

Fig. 71 Diagrammatic representation of the relationship between LV filling pressure and cardiac output. Treatment varies for patients in each quadrant (see text). CO = cardiac output. Pre-load = LV end-diastolic pressure.

expansion can be used in conjunction with inotropic agents (see also Fig. 57, p. 195). If cardiac output is satisfactory but filling pressure is high (right upper quadrant), venous dilatation with nitroglycerine may be possible, provided the patient is not frankly hypotensive. Where filling pressure is high but cardiac output is low (right lower quadrant), inotropic agents are indicated, possibly in conjunction with arterial, and sometimes venous, vasodilators. Although dramatic improvements have been documented in a sizeable number of patients with this approach, some units feel that widespread use of this invasive approach has not proved beneficial, and restrict use of the techniques to patients where there are specific problems in deciding about management.

Diuretics are the drugs of first choice for the treatment of cardiac failure due to acute myocardial infarction. Because of its rapid action, the best drug is frusemide given in a dose of 40 to 80 mg intravenously or orally. Digoxin should be used in chronic cardiac failure after infarction, particularly if the heart is enlarged, but its effect in acute infarction is disappointing and there is some evidence that it may increase infarct size. Acidosis, if present, is treated with bicarbonate. If inotropic support is required dopamine or dobutamine are most commonly used, rarely in doses greater than 5 μg per kg per min. Isoprenaline can be used but arrhythmias are more common with this agent and, particularly if tachycardia occurs, cardiac ischaemia can be worsened. Sodium nitroprusside can be used for combined arterial and venous dilatation, or nitroglycerine when venous dilatation is primarily required. Sometimes the use of oral agents is feasible, in which case commonly favoured drugs are prazosin and isosorbide dinitrate.

The frankly shocked patient is cold, pale and sweating with a systemic arterial pressure less than 90 mmHg. Confusion and oliguria denote reduced cerebral and renal blood flow. Treatment outlined above is utilised but only a small number of patients respond. Some units have investigated the use of balloon counter pulsation, with some success. Even in survivors, however, the death rate in the ensuing months has been disappointingly high and most units feel that this technique has very limited application.

A number of approaches have been tried in an attempt to limit infarct size. Some have been shown effective in experimental situations, but the variable severity of disease and time of presentation in patients has made confirmation difficult in the clinical situation. At present, early administration of beta receptor blocker drugs shows some promise.

The prevention of embolism

Since intravenous or intracardiac clotting is common after myocardial infarction, and embolism thus a serious risk, anticoagulant drugs are sometimes given to patients with acute infarction. Once widespread, this practice is now largely restricted to high risk patients, a history of previous thromboembolism, atrial fibrillation, low cardiac output, obesity and immobility being the primary indications. Treatment is started with intravenous heparin for 24 hr and continued with warfarin, according to Table 14.

Table 14 Dosage of anticoagulants.

	Initial dose	Maintenance dose	Controlling test
Heparin	5000 units IV	5000 units 4-hourly IV	Clotting time to 25–30 min
Warfarin	10–20 mg orally	3–10 mg daily	Prothrombin ratio 2 to 4

A close watch should be kept for bruising, haematuria or melaena in any patient receiving an anticoagulant. Passive and active limb movements are carried out frequently to discourage the formation of thrombi.

Rehabilitation and education

The rehabilitation programme starts when the patient enters the CCU. Both the patient and his family are usually extremely anxious. He has suffered a sudden change from a normal (or at least stable) health to a situation which is life-threatening. The patient and his family should know that staff recognise and sympathise with their anxieties. A quietly competent and confident manner, and an explanation of procedures in the CCU and prospects for the patient can do much to help in the initial period. The nature of the illness, its management and the healing process should be explained as soon as practicable, Sometimes a recorded tape is used to advantage to supplement individual explanation. The patient and his family must see him, from the earliest possible stage, as having an excellent chance of recovery and return to normal life; over 85 per cent of patients will achieve this. Obviously the approach to the critically ill, high risk patient, must be different. Although skill and tact are needed in handling this situation, honesty is essential.

If progress is uneventful the patient will increase his activities from the second or third day. He may feel insecure when monitoring is stopped but can be reassured that he no longer needs intensive care. Discharge from hospital is usually possible by the tenth day and, after discharge, the patient should continue to increase his exercise level daily. Provided symptoms are not intrusive it should be possible to walk a mile and to engage in sexual intercourse within 3 to 4 weeks, and to return to sedentary or light physical work in 4 to 5 weeks. Anxieties about convalescence should be anticipated and answered. Follow-up is required with the patient and his family to answer any questions, detect any complications, supervise treatment and ensure that convalescence is progressing satisfactorily. The Unit must work in close collaboration with the family practitioner. Abstaining from smoking and maintaining good control of blood pressure where required are most important features of management; achievement of ideal weight, a reasonable level of physical exercise, and treatment of hyperlipidaemia where present are also desirable. Therapy with a beta blocker is required in some cases and coronary arterial surgery is indicated for patients with persistent, severe angina, and those with lesser angina but with a markedly abnormal exercise electrocardiogram. Surgery is also required in some patients with arrhythmias or left ventricular failure associated with aneurysm formation.

Coronary-arterial surgery

In recent years the development of coronary-arterial surgery has produced a dramatic change in the prognosis of patients with severe angina.

The extent of atheroma is first demonstrated by cineangiography, in which radiographic contrast material is injected through special catheters into each coronary artery and its progress recorded as a motion picture. There may be many regions of important narrowing in the coronary arteries but, if these are proximal and the distal vessels are of reasonable calibre (1·5 mm or more) the obstructions can be satisfactorily bypassed by a graft leading directly from the aorta. The patient's saphenous vein is usually employed as the graft, but other veins or the internal mammary artery may be used. The operation requires cardiopulmonary bypass, several grafts may be inserted in one operation, and an infarct or aneurysm can be resected at the same time. With venous grafts, one end is anastomosed to the aorta and the other to the coronary artery, placing the graft so that blood flow is in the normal direction and there is thus no obstruction by venous valves.

Any patient in whom severe angina of effort persists, despite treatment with trinitrin, long-acting coronary dilators such as isosorbide dinitrate (Carvasin or Isordil) and beta-receptor blocking drugs, should be considered for operation. In suitable cases the operative risk is very low and relief from angina dramatic. Occasionally the distal coronary arteries are so severely affected by atheroma that grafting is impracticable but this is rare. Sometimes, too, the myocardium has been so destroyed by ischaemic damage that grafting is ineffective. Most patients, however, even those with fairly extensive infarction, benefit from coronary grafting, combined if necessary with excision of localised infarcts or aneurysms.

The indications for surgery in patients whose angina is not disabling are gradually becoming clearer. Patients with severe lesions of the left main coronary artery (75 to 90 per cent cross sectional area, Fig. 72) are at very high risk and require operation. Patients with triple vessel disease (i.e. disease in the region of the left anterior, left circumflex and right coronary arteries) are also at higher than usual risk, the precise level depending on the extent of disease in each area and the degree to which the left ventricle has been damaged. Patients with a severe proximal lesion of the left anterior descending coronary artery are also at increased risk, especially if there is associated occlusion of the right coronary artery. Marked ST depression or elevation, frequent ventricular premature beats or hypotension with exercise occur in many of the high risk patients and indicate those who need coronary arteriography with a view to surgery. Radio isotope studies with exercise add a further degree of precision to this assessment.

The place of coronary-arterial surgery in patients with recent myocardial infarction is not yet clearly established. In one or two aggressive units, all patients presenting with infarction are studied and submitted to urgent surgery. Except for patients with a very low cardiac output or shock, results of surgery are good. Few communities have the capacity to carry out such a programme and it is unlikely that this will become a widespread practice. Better returns are likely from a policy of education about risk factors and prevention, combined with selection of patients at high risk before infarction occurs. Attempts to salvage patients in shock, if necessary supporting them with balloon counter pulsation during preoperative investigation, have proved disappointing.

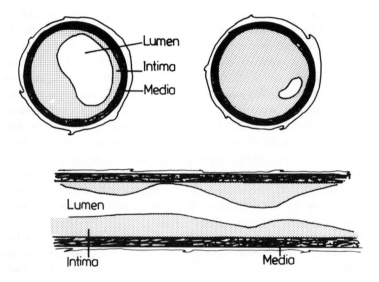

Fig. 72 Diagrammatic representation of a cross section of a coronary artery at two sites and the corresponding longitudinal section. The atheromatous lesion in the left-hand section occupies about 75 per cent of the cross sectional area (50 per cent of the diameter) and of the right-hand section 90 per cent of the cross sectional area (75 per cent of the diameter).

Another new approach is the infusion into the coronary artery of *streptokinase*. If this is infused at an early stage after infarction, any thrombus formed can be dissolved. This approach may have a particular place in the treatment of patients with proximal disease of the anterior descending coronary artery, which may be particularly hazardous. Subsequently, in suitable cases, the atheromatous lesion may be dealt with by *percutaneous transluminal angioplasty*. A special catheter with a balloon is placed under angiographic control and the balloon is inflated in a controlled way at the site of the narrowing. This technique has had an increasing application, particularly in patients with single major lesions. The atheromatous lesion becomes largely dispersed into the wall of the coronary and the narrowing is usually much improved. Facilities for immediate coronary surgery must be available when this technique is employed. Its role in the early stages of myocardial infarction is still under investigation.

The situation with patients who have severe and prolonged angina, but who have not progressed to infarction is different. Emergency coronary arteriography and operation can be undertaken in such patients with an acceptable risk, and impending infarction may be averted. The term 'pre-infarction angina' has been used to describe patients in whom unstable angina is thought likely to lead to infarction. The problem is to select patients who need operation because, in many with this clinical picture, symptoms subside spontaneously without the occurrence of infarction. Patients with prolonged anginal pain, with prominent ischaemic changes in the ECG and a long history of angina, appear most liable to infarction and should therefore be considered for urgent operation. Gross ST depression or elevation usually indicate proximal narrowing of an artery supplying a large area of myocardium. A less common indication is the presence of continued, life-threatening arrhythmias which may also be controlled by coronary-arterial grafting, sometimes combined with excision of an infarct or aneurysm. Electrophysiological studies are playing an increasing role in the management of such patients.

For the most part, postoperative management of patients undergoing coronary-arterial bypass grafting presents no special difficulty. It should, however, be noted that any persistent ischaemic region will remain unduly sensitive to the arrhythmogenic effect of isoprenaline. Although many patients need digoxin in the postoperative period, early problems with low cardiac output are uncommon except in patients with severe, preoperative damage to the left ventricle.

11   Respiratory Intensive Care

Respiratory care is based on four important principles:
1 The airway must be kept clear.
2 Alveolar ventilation must be adequate.
3 Arterial blood must be adequately oxygenated.
4 Pre-existing pulmonary disease must be treated and complications avoided.

1   Maintenance of a clear airway

The airway may be obstructed at any level. *Partial obstruction* of the big airways (trachea, main and lobar bronchi) increases the frictional work of breathing (p. 69) and, if severe or progressive, ultimately leads to exhaustion and ventilatory failure (p. 78). *Total obstruction* of the trachea causes rapid death from asphyxia. Obstruction of segmental and smaller bronchi and bronchioles causes uneven ventilation of alveoli, and in turn arterial hypoxia. Alveoli collapse beyond completely obstructed small bronchi, causing scattered opacities in the chest x-ray.

Acute airway obstruction can be rapidly fatal, especially in infants. Its recognition is thus vital. The following signs occur:
a Inspiratory and expiratory effort is increased.
b Breathing may be noisy—stridor in large airways, wheeze in small.
c The intercostal spaces are drawn in during inspiration.
d Respiratory frequency is variable but is usually increased in severe obstruction.
e When due to obstruction of the bigger airways, cyanosis is a late sign, and the diagnosis should be made before it develops.

Causes and treatment of airway obstruction

1 *Bronchial secretions* and inflammatory exudate are the most

241

common cause. They can be expelled by regular, assisted coughing but an abdominal or thoracic wound or injury may demand adequate relief from pain before coughing can become effective. Pain can usually be relieved by a narcotic drug such as papaveretum, but sometimes not without undue respiratory depression. Thoracic epidural block may then be of value. When cough is ineffective or absent, due to weakness or coma, aspiration of secretions through a tracheal tube or bronchoscope is necessary. Thick, sticky sputum is hard to cough up and so the patient must be adequately hydrated to prevent the drying and crusting of sputum.

2   In unconscious or very weak patients *the tongue* tends to fall back and occlude the airway. This is prevented by nursing the patient on his side and by inserting an oropharyngeal airway.

3   Patients who are unconscious or weak, or who have difficulty in swallowing due to myasthenia or bulbar paralysis, are constantly at risk of *inhaling foreign material*. When vomit is inhaled, gastric acid causes oedema of the airway, bronchiolar spasm, alveolar oedema and pneumonia. The risk of inhalation of vomit is much reduced by nursing the patient head down on his side; a deeply unconscious patient should have his trachea intubated until protective reflexes return. Tracheostomy may be necessary for long-term isolation of the airway from the pharynx.

4   *Oedema of the airway* may be due to infection (especially in children), to allergic reactions, or to irritation by a tracheal tube, removal of which is then followed by obstruction. Adrenaline (p. 32) steroids (p. 134) and/or urgent intubation may be required.

5   *A tracheal tube* does not guarantee a clear airway. It may be compressed, kinked or blocked by encrusted sputum. The cuff may bulge over the end of the tube. If a tube seems to be obstructed the cuff should be deflated and manual ventilation with oxygen attempted. If manual ventilation is not possible the tube is obstructed and needs urgent repositioning or removal. If the tube is removed ventilation is continued via a face mask or the tracheostomy stoma until the tube is replaced. Alternatively, if oxygen passes easily down the tube and escapes past the deflated cuff, the latter may have been the cause of the obstruction. Tube patency should be confirmed by passage of a suction catheter, and the cuff re-inflated with a smaller volume. If manual ventilation remains impossible after tube replacement the most likely causes are tracheal or bronchial obstruction due to secretions, blood clot or extrinsic pressure.

Severe bronchospasm or tension pneumothorax, can also make ventilation very difficult.

Tracheal intubation

A tube may be passed into the trachea through the mouth (oro-tracheal), through the nose (nasotracheal) or through a surgical opening in the tracheal wall (tracheostomy). The choice depends on circumstances and upon the practice of the Intensive Care Unit. In general, intubation for less than 3 days does not call for tracheostomy.

Indications

1 To relieve obstruction of the upper part of the airway.
2 To allow aspiration of sputum which the patient cannot cough up.
3 To safeguard the airway from foreign matter when swallowing and/or coughing are impaired.
4 To allow IPPV or CPAP to be carried out.

Care of a patient with a tracheal tube

1 Whenever possible the procedure should first be explained to the patient. He should know that the tube will prevent speech. The following items should be readily available:
a A pencil, paper and firm writing surface by means of which the patient may communicate.
b An efficient suction pump and tube ending in a plastic or metal Y-piece.
c Sterile suction catheters.
d A spare tracheal tube of the same size as that in place, a laryngoscope and (if a tracheostomy has been done) a tracheostomy dilator.
e A 10-ml syringe for inflating the cuff of the tracheal tube.
f A humidifier.
g Means of manual ventilation, e.g. an Ambu bag, ready fitted with connectors to match the tracheal tube. A facemask should also be provided lest removal of a faulty tube be necessary.
h A device (e.g. Wright 'Respirometer') for measuring tidal volume and ventilation.

2 *Removal of secretions.* A tracheal tube, which is a foreign body, increases the bronchial secretion-rate above normal, and since effective coughing is impossible this sputum must be aspirated without injuring or infecting the delicate lining of the airway. Pulmonary disease may add to the volume of sputum to be cleared.

a *'Artificial coughing'.* An intubated patient cannot close his vocal cords to build up the pressure necessary for a normal cough, and secretions in the smaller airways cannot be properly dislodged. However, by posturing each lung uppermost in turn, and with manual inflation followed by firm compression of rib cage and abdomen together, distal secretions can be squeezed (like toothpaste!) into the medium-sized bronchi. Once there they can usually be coughed within reach of an aspirating catheter. The manoeuvre is often called 'artificial coughing', but it must be understood that it cannot compare in efficiency with a natural cough.

b *Aspiration* is indicated: if sputum can be heard rattling in the trachea, before and after turning the patient from one side to the other (usually done every 2 hours), before and after deflating the cuff of the tube, and if the patient requests it.

Suction catheters should be soft and pliable, have both end and side holes, and be less than half the inside diameter of the tracheal tube. If the tip of the catheter is angulated it can be directed into either the left or right main bronchus (a straight catheter goes most often down the right main bronchus). A means of controlling the suction must be incorporated in the system, the most convenient being a Y-piece or side hole in the suction line which can be occluded with the thumb to initiate suction. Aseptic technique is desirable and sterile suction catheters should not be touched with the bare hands. Isotonic saline solution ($0 \cdot 1$ ml/kg) instilled into the tracheal tube before aspiration may help to remove tenacious secretions. The suction catheter is passed down the tracheal tube as far as it will go, suction is then applied and the catheter withdrawn with a rotary motion. Prolonged suction causes hypoxia and the procedure should be limited to 15 to 20 seconds. Each catheter is discarded after use. Suction is usually applied during withdrawal of the catheter, but, if it is suspected that a large amount of secretion is present in either the trachea or the tracheal tube, it is worth applying suction while the catheter is being introduced, provided the suction is released immediately the catheter becomes obstructed. This technique is called dunking, and prevents secretions being pushed down the trachea. Negative pressure in the airways may cause small areas of atelectasis and most units advocate a few manual hyperinflations of the lungs after tracheal aspiration in order to re-expand these areas. Aspiration is easier if an assistant is available, and, assistance may be essential in dealing with infants.

3 *Humidification.* A tracheal tube bypasses the upper airway which normally warms and moistens inspired air (p. 75). This function is thus transferred to the lower airway which becomes inflamed and encrusted with dry secretions. The action of cilia decreases when the inspired air is less than 75 per cent saturated with water at 37°C or when the temperature of the inspired air is above 41°C. These problems can be prevented by humidifying the air artificially. Ideally, air entering the tracheal tube should be fully saturated with water vapour at body temperature. Two methods of humidification are available:

a *Hot water humidification* in which air is blown over water whose temperature is thermostatically controlled. For an adult breathing by himself an air flow of at least 20 litres per min is necessary. A temperature of 32°C at the tracheal tube ensures 75 per cent saturation by the time the air reaches the alveolae. In practice the thermostat is set to secure a tempertature of 35 to 37°C at the tracheal tube to ensure adequate humidification without the danger of scalding the trachea.

b *Nebulization*, in which water is dispersed through the inspired gas as minute droplets. Humidification can be far greater than in method **a**, but the gas is not warmed in most instruments and this is a disadvantage. Bronchodilator drugs (p. 34) can be added to many of the available nebulizers.

4 *Care of the tracheal tube.* Movement of the tube within the trachea quickly causes abrasion, ulceration and infection. The tube must therefore be firmly fixed by adhesive strapping, tape or elastic. The cuff, if there is one, must be inflated with just enough air to prevent the escape of inspired air around it, when used with a respirator, or expired air around it with the mouth of the tube occluded, when not used with a respirator. Overinflation of the cuff predisposes to ulceration of the trachea, to herniation of the cuff and to difficulty in swallowing.

The advent of low pressure cuffs has rendered regular deflation of the cuff unnecessary, but high pressure cuffs should be regularly deflated to allow circulation of the trachael lining to recover. Cuffed tubes are never used in infants or small children.

A tracheostomy calls for special care of the surrounding skin. Dry gauze should be frequently changed under the flange of the tracheostomy tube. In some units the area is sprayed with neomycin-bacitracin-polmyxin powder. Great care must be taken to prevent inhalation of the spray. The elastic or tape retaining the tracheostomy tube may easily ulcerate the skin round the neck unless it is suitably padded.

5 *Complications of tracheal intubation* (Fig. 73). Almost all the following can be avoided by scrupulous nursing care:

a *Tracheal injury* may result from excessive movement of the tube, overinflation of the cuff and clumsy use of suction-catheters. The ulceration and infection, so caused, greatly impede recovery and may lead to permanent tracheal stenosis.

b *Blockage of the tube* by crusted secretions follows inadequate humidification, and herniation of the cuff (p. 242) may occlude the end of the tube.

c *Pulmonary infection* is favoured by poor humidification, poor aspiration technique and inadequate physiotherapy. Humidifiers must be cleaned, sterilized and refilled frequently, and always before use with another patient.

d *Pulmonary collapse* follows inadequate aspiration. It also occurs if the tube, being too long, protrudes into one or other main bronchus, usually the right; this is recognized by the diminution or absence of breath sounds over the other lung.

2 Maintenance of adequate alveolar ventilation

Ventilatory failure exists when the alveolar ventilation is insufficient to meet the need for gas exchange at a normal level of $P\text{CO}_2$ in the arterial blood. Its causes have been summarized (p. 87). It may occur (a) when the lungs are normal but alveolar ventilation is too low, or (b) in lung disease, when alveolar ventilation is low, normal or even above normal; in this case uneven distribution of inspired gas (p. 76) leads to uneconomical use of the available ventilation. In all cases the arterial blood $P\text{CO}_2$ is the standard by which the adequacy of ventilation is judged. The proper ventilation is that which avoids an abnormally high or low $P\text{CO}_2$ (above 6 kPa (45 mmHg) or below 4 kPa (30 mmHg)).

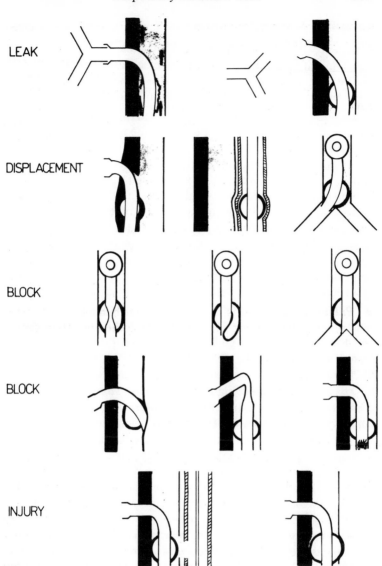

Fig. 73 Some complications of tracheal intubation: (*top row*) ruptured cuff, disconnection; (*2nd row*) tube in subcutaneous tissue, oesophagus, bronchus (anterior view); (*3rd and 4th rows*) tube blocked by compression, bulging cuff, impaction on carina, displacement, kinking, secretion and (*bottom row*) fistula, overdistended cuff.

Recognition of ventilatory failure

A patient with ventilatory failure is hypercapnic (raised arterial P_{CO_2}) and, if breathing air, is also hypoxic (low arterial P_{O_2}). The clincial signs of ventilatory failure are due to these changes in blood gases and to the attempts of the body to correct them.

a   *Hypercapnia.* CO_2 dilates arterioles and capillaries directly, and also stimulates the sympathetic centre in the brain leading to a rise in cardiac output. At first the increased cardiac output predominates, and the patient has a raised blood pressure with a warm skin and a full pulse. When P_{CO_2} is very high (more than 10 kPa or 80 mmHg), CO_2 becomes a central depressant; the patient becomes drowsy and confused. Owing to dilation of cerebral arterioles, blood flow through the brain increases and intracranial pressure rises, and the patient may complain of headache. Convulsions may occur. At still higher levels the vasomotor centre begins to be depressed and blood pressure falls.

It is important to note that when breathing air the arterial P_{CO_2} seldom reaches 13 kPa (about 100 mmHg) because the accompanying hypoxia would otherwise be fatal. When the patient is breathing O_2 the P_{CO_2} may rise much higher and the signs of central depression are then seen. Hypercapnia is not nearly as dangerous as hypoxia.

b   *Hypoxia.* The direct sign of hypoxia is *cyanosis*, in this case *central cyanosis* (p. 83). In ventilatory failure uncomplicated by any condition causing shock (p. 192) the cyanosis is usually obvious in the blueness of the skin, mouth and nailbeds. This is because the accompanying hypercapnia dilates the superficial vessels and these are full of blood. Cyanosis may then be detectable at an arterial saturation of between 80 and 85 per cent and obvious below 75 per cent. On the other hand, when superficial vessels are almost empty, as in shock, cyanosis may be missed even when severe arterial hypoxia is present. The haemoglobin concentration of the blood also affects the appearance of cyanosis. It may be obvious in polycythaemia and very difficult to detect in anaemic states. In severe anaemia there may not be enough reduced haemoglobin to give a blue colour.

The other signs of hypoxia are less definite. By central stimulation, arterioles constrict and cardiac output increases, *raising the blood pressure*; but if hypoxia impairs cardiac performance, *output and pressure may fall. Anxiety, restlessness and confusion*, in order of development, are common indications of hypoxia but may be mistaken for the similar effects of hypercapnia if this is present. Worse still, these signs may be attributed to pain, or to 'hangover' from anaesthetic or sedatives, or to the effects of cerebral vascular disease, all of which might reasonably indicate further sedation; in fact the patient needs ventilating, or oxygen, or both. *In these circumstances a sedative or narcotic drug by itself can only make hypoxia worse by depressing ventilation still more.*

c *Signs arising from attempts of the body to correct hypercapnia and hypoxia.* A rise in PCO_2 is normally a powerful stimulus to breathing, and a fall in PO_2, if marked, also increases ventilation (p. 75). The increased ventilatory stimulus shows itself clinically by a rising respiratory frequency and by evidence, detectable by careful observation, of increased inspiratory effort. The accessory muscles of inspiration (p. 72) are increasingly active, and a tell-tale sign is often the widening of the nostrils which these patients may show with each breath. This clinical picture is well seen in advancing polyneuritis with respiratory paralysis, and by the time it appears the patient is extensively paralysed.

On the other hand, evidence of increased ventilatory effort may not be obvious, or indeed present at all, if the respiratory centre or respiratory muscles are not capable of responding to the raised PCO_2. This is seen especially in the late stages of chronic bronchitis and emphysema. These patients gradually lose the ability to respond to a rise in PCO_2 by increasing ventilation, and their breathing becomes more and more dependent upon the hypoxic stimulus (p. 75). If this stimulus is removed by breathing a high concentration of O_2, serious underventilation may ensue and the already high PCO_2 becomes even higher. Insensitivity to CO_2 is seldom important unless arterial PCO_2 has been persistently high for some time. Whenever O_2 is given to such a patient he should be closely watched for evidence of increasing hypercapnia.

Treatment aims at increasing alveolar ventilation to an adequate level.

1 Gross abnormalities which reduce effective ventilation must be corrected if possible. Airway obstruction is one example (p. 241), and asthmatic obstruction calls for special measures (p. 262). Pneumothorax, haemothorax and pleural effusion must be dealt with (p. 182).

2   Drugs which depress breathing, and high O_2 concentrations in patients with depressed CO_2 response, should be avoided in patients not artificially ventilated. Once ventilation has been taken over mechanically these restrictions do not necessarily apply.

3   Respiratory stimulants have a limited place in treatment. The continuous intravenous infusion of *nikethamide* at 5 to 10 mg per min is of some value in patients with advanced chronic pulmonary disease in whom intubation and IPPV are often best avoided. Nikethamide can produce a worthwhile increase in ventilation, and (perhaps more importantly) arousal of a stuporose patient who thus co-operates more effectively in supervised coughing. Other stimulants, e.g. dichlorphenamide, are of doubtful value.

4   Although the decision to start IPPV may not have been taken, it is sometimes useful to pass a tracheal tube so that the airway can be thoroughly aspirated and the lungs well inflated a few times by Ambu bag.

5   Patients with ventilatory failure quickly become dehydrated unless careful attention is given to water and electrolyte balance. Dehydration renders secretions sticky and hard to cough up or aspirate. Intravenous fluids are usually indicated to prevent this.

6   Should the above treatment fail to produce the desired result, and provided the cause of the ventilatory failure is considered reversible (p. 265), intermittent positive pressure ventilation is begun.

Intermittent positive-pressure ventilation (IPPV)

Artificial ventilation is used to provide an adequate alveolar ventilation when other means have failed, and/or to reduce (or abolish) the patient's respiratory work (p. 71). In emergency, mouth-to-mouth resuscitation can be carried out, or the patient can be manually ventilated with bag and mask. For prolonged artificial ventilation tracheal intubation and a mechanical ventilator are needed.

Mechanical ventilators. There are so many different makes that a full account will not be given here. ICU staff should take pains to become thoroughly familiar with the type of machine they use. Ventilators can be classified according to the mechanism of generating the inspiratory flow, and from the mode of cycling (Table 15). Depending on the combination of these variables, the machine will

Table 15 Functional classification of ventilators.

Primary classification depends on driving mechanism	Subclassification depends on the method used to cycle the machine	
	Method used to initiate inspiration	Method used to initiate expiration
	1 Time from the previous inspiration	1 Time of inspiration
Pressure generator	2 Volume expired	2 Volume inspired
	3 Airway pressure at end-expiration	3 Airway pressure at end-inspiration
Flow generator	4 Flow at end-expiration	4 Flow at end-inspiration
	5 Patient inspiratory effort	5 Other
	6 Other	

deliver either a preset volume or a preset pressure with each inspiration.

1 *Volume preset ventilators* (e.g. Engstrom, Bennett MA 1 & 2, Cape) deliver a constant volume at each inspiration. This volume is not changed by changes in lung compliance or airway resistance and the pressure reached during inspiration depends on these two factors. If an obstruction develops in the lower airway a dangerously high pressure may develop. Some machines have a safety mechanism which prevents this and all modern ones have an alarm to indicate when it happens.

2 *Pressure preset ventilators* (e.g. Bird, Bennett PR-2) provide an inspiratory flow until a preset airway pressure is reached, regardless of the volume which has been delivered. If compliance falls or resistance increases, the inspiratory volume falls. Many modern machines can be used as either volume preset or pressure preset ventilators.

The start of each inspiration may be set to occur after a desired interval (time cycled) or inspiration can be triggered by the patient's own respiratory effort (patient cycled). The latter is useful when, as is usually the case, spontaneous respiratory activity is present and the patient needs only assistance from the ventilator.

Ongoing assessment during IPPV. The following details should be recorded regularly, usually every half hour. A marked change at any time or a trend over a period of time may mean the treatment should be altered.

1 *Respiratory frequency* should remain constant, for any given setting, if ventilation is entirely controlled. When the patient's inspiration is used to trigger the ventilator, frequency is affected by all the factors which apply in spontaneous breathing (p. 76).

2 *Tidal volume* should be constant if the machine is volume-cycled. A fall in volume suggests the presence of a leak, which may be due to an under-inflated or burst cuff, or to a loose connection anywhere between the tracheal tube and the ventilator. With a pressure-cycled machine an increase in tidal volume suggests that pulmonary compliance has improved, while a fall indicates either airway obstruction or reduced compliance. Tidal volume is measured with a meter such as the Wright Respirometer, at the *expiratory* port of the ventilator. This ensures that only gas which has actually entered and left the patient's lungs is measured.

3 Expired volume should be measured over 1 min to give the *ventilation rate*, and then divided by respiratory frequency to obtain the average tidal volume. For an adult, a tidal volume of 8 to 10 ml per kg and a frequency of 10 to 16 breaths per min, with pulmonary ventilation of 80 to 120 ml per kg per min, are usually adequate.

4 *The peak inflation-pressure* (inspiratory pressure) should ideally be measured near to the tracheal tube, to reflect true airway pressure most closely. However, in many ventilators, the manometer (pressure meter) is part of the machine, and the resistance of the ventilator tubing affects the reading. In a pressure-preset machine, the cut-off pressure is set to provide an adequate tidal volume. The stiffer the lungs, the higher the pressure needed. In a volume-preset ventilator, inflation pressure is recorded because it gives information about pulmonary compliance or obstruction. *A rise in inflation pressure* indicates stiffening of the lungs (fall in compliance) due to atelectasis, pneumonia or oedema, or to obstruction somewhere between the pressure meter and the alveoli; this may be in the ventilator tubing, the tracheal tube or the airway. *A fall in inflation* *pressure* may denote improved compliance but may also be due to a leak; this must be excluded carefully.

5 *Inspired O₂ concentration* may have to be changed according to the arterial PO_2 and it should be regularly measured with an oxygen analyser.

Management of a patient during IPPV

All the nursing procedures for a patient with a tracheal tube apply.

Ward preparation. In addition to the preparations described on p. 243 the selected ventilator should be connected to its power supply and tested for leaks. The humidifier should be filled with sterile, distilled water and warmed to the appropriate temperature. Suitable connections from the ventilator to the tracheal tube should be assembled and a means of manual ventilation must be at hand.

Operation of the ventilator

1 *A patient who is apnoeic* is usually easily controlled. The ventilator is set for automatic operation at the desired frequency and tidal volume. Inspiration should occupy about ¹/₃ of the respiratory cycle. The volume and frequency should be altered if measurement of arterial PCO_2 shows that alveolar ventilation is not satisfactory (p. 87).

2 *A patient who is still breathing* can almost always be induced to accept patient-triggered ventilatory assistance, provided that the airway is clear and alveolar ventilation adequate. In the initial stages, small doses (5 mg) of papaveretum or diazepam will help the patient to become accustomed to ventilatory assistance and prevent him from 'fighting the respirator'. The machine should be set so that automatic operation begins if the patient's inspiratory effort becomes too weak to trigger it.

Other aspects of management

1 *Water and electrolyte balance.* Even mild dehydration is dangerous for an intubated patient. IPPV exaggerates the increase in secretion of aldosterone and ADH which occurs in the postoperative period (p. 24). An accurate record of water, sodium and potassium balance must be kept and the patient's needs calculated and supplied.

2 *Nutrition.* Intravenous infusion of 5 per cent glucose solution can provide, at most, 150 g of glucose, equivalent to $150 \times 4 = 600$ Cal (2 510 kJ), daily. It is thus essential to give more carbohydrate, as well as fat and protein, as soon as intestinal function permits. Since a naso-tracheal or orotracheal tube interferes with swallowing, the food must be homogenized and given through a nasogastric tube. In patients needing prolonged IPPV a tracheostomy is done, and these patients learn to swallow ordinary soft foods; a diet containing 80 g of protein, with added iron and vitamins and providing at least 2500 Calories (10 460 kJ), should be given. If renal failure is present, protein may have to be restricted.

3 *Antibiotics* should not be given unless there is clear evidence of infection, such as purulent tracheal aspirate, leucocytosis and fever.

4 *Supportive care.* The patient's morale is most important, and much can be done to minimize the psychological injury of distressing and sometimes prolonged illness. It must never be assumed that because a patient cannot speak he is deaf, confused or insensitive. All procedures should be gently explained in advance, and anything said in the patient's hearing must be circumspect. Care of pressure areas, regular turning from side to side, oral hygiene, and maximal active and passive limb movements must all receive attention.

Finally, a patient who is being mechanically ventilated *must never be left unattended.*

Assessment of progress. This is based, in general, upon the following observations: (a) arterial blood-gas and pH measurement, (b) trends in heart rate, arterial blood pressure, respiratory frequency, tidal volume and inflation pressure, (c) the quantity and appearance of material aspirated from the trachea, and the results of its thrice-weekly culture, and (d) clinical examination and x-rays of the chest at regular intervals.

Return to spontaneous breathing. When signs of recovery appear, the patient must be weaned from the ventilator. This may be a rapid or gradual procedure, depending on the nature of the original disorder, the duration of IPPV and the patient's overall clinical state. Rapid weaning is usually possible if IPPV was started for a non-respiratory reason and has not been prolonged, e.g. elective ventilation of under 48 hr after major surgery. In the presence of chronic lung disease, or after long ventilation, gradual weaning is usually required.

A start is made by disconnecting the ventilator and carefully following the patient's tidal volume, ventilation rate and respiratory frequency, while watching closely for signs of exhaustion, dyspnoea or cyanosis. After 30 to 60 min of spontaneous breathing, if all seems well, the arterial blood PO_2 and PCO_2 may be measured. If these too are satisfactory, it is usually possible to remove the tracheal tube forthwith. Some patients will falter at some point in this procedure and need a further spell of mechanical ventilation.

Gradual weaning may also be accomplished by the use of intermittent mandatory ventilation (IMV). In this technique the ventilator is set so that spontaneous breathing is augmented by a breath from the ventilator at preset intervals. These intervals are progressively increased over a period of hours or days until the patient is no longer dependent on the breaths from the machine.

Complications of IPPV

1 *Reduction of cardiac output.* The mean intrathoracic pressure is increased by IPPV (p. 73) especially when inflation pressure is high, inspiration prolonged unduly, or expiration impeded for any reason. This impedes the return of venous blood to the heart and lowers cardiac output and arterial pressure. A patient with normal cardiovascular reflexes compensates via the baroreceptor reflex by (a) venous constriction and sympathetic stimulation of the heart, maintaining cardiac output; and (b) arteriolar constriction, maintaining arterial pressure. When the compensatory mechanism is impaired, either because these adjustments are already maximal or for some other reason such as loss of blood, or because the sympathetic impulses to the arterioles and veins are blocked by polyneuritis or an α-blocking drug, the cardiac output and arterial pressure may fall sharply when IPPV is begun. When this happens, infusion of blood or plasma may increase venous pressure enough to restore an adequate cardiac output (p. 46).

2 *Mismatching of alveolar ventilation and blood flow* (p. 75). This always happens with IPPV, but is not serious unless there is already severe mismatching due to pulmonary disease. It shows

itself by the relatively high ventilation needed to keep arterial P_{CO_2} normal, and by the presence of some degree of hypoxia at normal P_{CO_2}.

3 *Alveolar collapse* is apt to occur during IPPV because of retained secretions and closure of small airways, a tendency which is aggravated if tidal volume remains constant for long periods. This complication must be prevented by thorough and frequent tracheal aspiration and by periodically giving a few deep breaths. Most modern ventilators have a mechanism that does this automatically. Application of a positive pressure at the expiratory valve ('positive end-expiratory pressure' or PEEP) may prevent the closure of small airways. However, PEEP further increases the mean intrathoracic pressure and may reduce cardiac output.

4 *Pulmonary infection* is favoured by IPPV and by the complication of alveolar collapse.

5 *Pneumothorax* is especially likely to occur if airway obstruction is present and a high inflation pressure is unavoidable, but it can happen in any patient having IPPV and can be quickly fatal if unrecognized and untreated. The most useful sign is dimunition or absence of expansion, during inspiration, of the affected side of the chest. Treatment is described on p. 265.

3   Maintenance of arterial oxygenation

The causes of hypoxia have been listed (p. 88). Its treatment follows logically from the particular mechanism concerned in each case. Taking the causes listed on p. 88 in turn:

1 *Reduction in inspired P_{O_2}* is relevant to clinical medicine only where the oxygen supply has been wrongly connected. This does happen, and it is wise always to check that connections (including central connections in the case of a wall supply) have been correctly made.

2 *Underventilation of the alveoli* calls for measures to increase ventilation, usually by IPPV. This corrects the accompanying hypercapnia as well as the hypoxia. It would be wrong to relieve the hypoxia by oxygen therapy alone, for this would not improve the hypercapnia and might make it worse.

3 *Pulmonary disease* with mismatching of alveolar ventilation and blood flow, *if the hypoxia is not accompanied by a high arterial P_{CO_2},* requires oxygen therapy, with or without continuous positive airways pressure. If the arterial PCO_2 is increased, this indicates that overall alveolar ventilation is inadequate and IPPV will be necessary in addition to oxygen.

Occasionally, in disease of the lung, there is a barrier to transfer of O_2 from alveoli to capillaries, owing to thickening of alveolar walls. The transfer of CO_2 is *not* similarly affected. In the ICU such a 'diffusion' problem is rarely the only cause of a low arterial PO_2.

4   The hypoxia due to *shunting of blood from venous to arterial channels* arises because the shunted blood cannot pass through ventilated alveoli. It might be thought, therefore, that neither increasing ventilation nor the inhalation of high O_2 concentrations would improve the hypoxia. In fact, if 100 per cent O_2 is breathed, the arterial PO_2 may be kept near 13 kPa (about 100 mmHg) provided not more than one quarter of the cardiac output is shunted. The reason for this is that blood which passes through the capillaries of ventilated alveoli is able to take an extra load of oxygen in solution (p. 80); this extra oxygen is then available to oxygenate shunted blood further downstream.

Continuous positive pressure respiration

An important cause of mismatching of alveolar ventilation and blood flow, and thus of hypoxia, is closure of smaller bronchi and collapse of their distal alveolic atelectasis, p. 78).

After operation breathing tends to be shallow and cough ineffective because of tissue oedema, pain or the depressant effects of pain-relieving drugs, and atelectasis is thus common. Hypoxia will be especially marked in patients suffering from lung conditions which cause mismatching of alveolar ventilation and blood flow, e.g. pneumonia, pulmonary venous congestion and pulmonary oedema. The application of a continuous positive pressure to the airway, whether during spontaneous breathing (CPAP) or during artificial ventilation (PEEP), can overcome atelectasis or at least halt its progress.

Continuous positive airways pressure may be used:

1   To prevent or treat postoperative atelectasis, especially in infants (p. 280).

2   To improve oxygenation when oxygen therapy by mask fails to achieve a safe arterial PO_2.

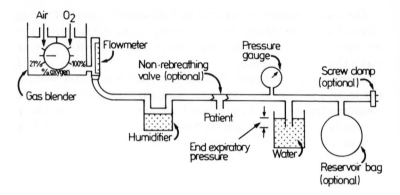

Fig. 74 Diagram of the arrangement for applying continuous positive airways pressure (CPAP). See text for explanation.

3 To wean a patient from IPPV when, with spontaneous breathing, the arterial $P\text{CO}_2$ is normal but the arterial $P\text{O}_2$ is low.

Fig. 74 shows the CPAP circuit. Humidified, warmed air and oxygen are delivered to the patient through an endotracheal tube. The positive pressure in the circuit depends on the depth that the wide-bore expiratory tube is placed underwater and is confirmed on the pressure gauge. An elastic reservoir bag in either the inspiratory or expiratory tubing reduces pressure fluctuations but this is unnecessary if a high gas flow is used. The gas flow should be at least three times the pulmonary ventilation to prevent rebreathing and a fall in airway pressure during inspiration. In practice, this is ensured by adjusting the flow so that the underwater valve is still bubbling during inspiration. An alternative method of generating the positive pressure uses a screw clamp on the expiratory tubing. In this case a reservoir bag must be incorporated and the underwater valve is set at a higher pressure (i.e. 30 cm H_2O) and acts purely as a safety valve to prevent accidental pressure build-up. The underwater safety valve should always be in the expiratory side of the circuit so that circuit deadspace does not increase when it operates. Although it is easier to set up, this screw clamp method is inferior as it does not accommodate to changes in gas flow, and pressure fluctuations with respiration are large especially when the patient takes a deep breath.

The initial positive end-expiratory pressure is usually set at 5 to 12 cm H_2O and the inspired oxygen at 70 to 80 per cent. Blood gases are measured at frequent intervals and an arterial PO_2 not less than 9 kPa (70 mmHg) is aimed at. If the arterial PO_2 is greater than 11 kPa (80 mmHg) the inspired oxygen is reduced in a stepwise manner to 40 per cent while the positive inspiratory pressure is held constant. When arterial PO_2 is adequate with an inspired oxygen concentration of 40 per cent, the CPAP is gradually reduced. The patient is then usually ready for extubation.

Oxygen therapy

Mechanism of action. When pure O_2 is breathed, the nitrogen in ventilated alveoli, ordinarily about 80 per cent of the alveolar gas, is gradually washed out and its place taken by O_2. Alveolar PO_2 thus increases from 13 to about 85 kPa (100 to 650 mmHg). A smaller increase results when air-O_2 mixtures are breathed.

Indications. The basic reason for giving oxygen is to relieve *tissue hypoxia*, when this is of a type which can be relieved. The causes of tissue hypoxia are as follows:
1 *Reduction in the oxygenation of arterial blood*: this has just been discussed and is also dealt with on p. 82.
2 *Reduction in blood flow to the tissues.* Normal oxygenation of arterial blood is of no value to tissues which do not receive any blood, and is of limited value to those which have a reduced blood supply. A reduction in blood flow may be generalized, i.e. when the *cardiac output is low.* Although blood oxygenation may be normal breathing air, it is possible to increase the dissolved O_2 in arterial blood by breathing a high concentration of O_2, and thus increase the amount of O_2 delivered to the tissues. The extra benefit is small, but may be of great value in severe shock. When reduction of blood flow is localized, as in *arterial obstruction*, oxygen therapy is less consistently useful but may be indicated in certain cases.
3 Tissue hypoxia may also result, despite a normal PO_2 in arterial blood, when the *concentration of available haemoglobin* is reduced. This may happen in *anaemia* and also when part of the haemoglobin is made unavailable, as in *carbon monoxide poisoning*. In the latter, O_2 therapy is valuable because it helps to displace carbon monoxide from its combination with haemoglobin. In anaemia, O_2 therapy

may help by increasing dissolved O_2, but blood transfusion is more direct and effective.

4 Finally, even with normal oxygenation of arterial blood, a normal haemoglobin level and a normal blood supply, the tissues may become hypoxic because they *cannot utilize the oxygen* they receive. This happens in cyanide poisoning, which is rarely seen but may occur during nitroprusside infusion (p. 119) and in which O_2 therapy is naturally valueless.

The sections on *recognition of hypoxia* (p. 248) and *cyanosis* should be revised in connection with this account of O_2 therapy.

Method of administration

1 *Masks.* If oxygen is supplied to a mask at a rate higher than the *maximal* rate at which the patient inspires from the mask then nothing but O_2 can be breathed; the excess O_2 will escape through the holes in the mask. The maximal inspiratory flow rate is about three times the pulmonary ventilation. For a patient breathing at 6 to 7 l per min, the maximal inspiratory flow would be about 20 l per min. To supply O_2 to the mask at or above this rate would be wasteful, and lower rates are almost always used. In this case, however, it must be accepted that for part of the respiratory cycle the patient is breathing in from the mask faster than O_2 is being supplied to it. The inspired O_2, during this phase, is diluted with gas already in the mask (which may contain some CO_2 expired in the previous breath) and also with room air sucked in through holes in the mask. On average, therefore, the patient is breathing less than 100 per cent O_2, and the lower the O_2 flows the lower will be the average O_2 concentration inspired. He will also be rebreathing some of his expired CO_2, and again this effect will be greater the lower the flow of O_2 into the mask.

It is essential to grasp the above facts in order to understand the behaviour of various masks and what can be expected from them. They are of many kinds but fall broadly into two categories:

a *Those intended to provide high O_2 concentrations*, e.g. the Mary Catterall mask. Oxygen is fed to the mask at 4 to 8 l per min, giving O_2 concentrations of 35 to 65 per cent in the inspired air, depending on the patient's ventilation; the lower the ventilation, the higher the O_2 concentration, and if ventilation is very low the concentration may rise to 80 or 90 per cent. Rebreathing of CO_2 occurs, especially with the pliable 'Polymask'. The oxygen delivered to the mask should be humidified if it is used for long periods.

b *Those intended to provide air 'enriched' with O_2*, i.e. O_2 concentrations of 27 to 32 per cent. Examples are the 'Ventimask' and the 'Edinburgh Mask'. Since most of the inspired mixture is room air, oxygen need not be humidified. These masks, if properly used, do not allow rebreathing of expired CO_2.

2 *Catheters*. One or two soft catheters may be passed through the nostrils until their tips lie just below the soft palate, and O_2 may be supplied through these. A total flow of more than 2 l per min is not easily tolerated, but this gives effective O_2 concentrations of up to 50 per cent, depending on ventilation. Some patients tend to swallow a lot of gas. The oxygen must be humidified to avoid drying of the nasopharynx.

3 *Head boxes* are useful especially for infants and children. Made of clear rigid plastic, they enclose the head and neck while oxygen or oxygen-air mixtures can be fed into them, escaping through a wide hole at the top of the box. Unless flow is quite fast, rebreathing of CO_2 can be a problem. Head boxes are most appropriate when it is desired to give O_2-enriched air at high humidity.

4 *Tents* are less often used nowadays but can still be useful for restless patients who will not keep a mask or hood in place. Disadvantages are the high expenditure of O_2, the necessity to cool the contents of a tent to prevent rapid increase in temperature, the awkwardness of access, the certainty of big leaks whenever access is needed, and the danger of fire and explosion.

5 *CPAP* (p. 257).

6 *Ventilators* can be operated with air, oxygen, or air-oxygen mixtures. The range of concentrations of the mixture varies from one ventilator to another, and in many the concentration is apt to vary even when the setting is held constant. In some ventilators it is possible to adjust the setting to keep inspired concentration of O_2 constant. *In all O_2 therapy it is most desirable to monitor the inspired O_2 concentration with an O_2 analyser.*

Oxygen toxicity

Oxygen is poisonous when a high concentration is breathed for a long time.

1 Oxygen is *toxic to the lining of the bronchi and alveoli.*

Congestion, haemorrhage, oedema and exudation occur, and in severe cases the alveoli become filled with exudate, leading to decreased lung compliance and hypoxia. Oxygenation becomes progressively more difficult and death often results. It is often difficult to distinguish these changes from complications of the pulmonary disease for which O_2 was originally required.

The changes of *pulmonary oxygen toxicity*, as it is called, can occur after as little as 24 hours' breathing of 100 per cent O_2, but usually the interval is longer. Even 50 per cent O_2 carries some danger. It is thus very desirable to limit O_2 therapy wherever possible and to use the lowest concentration which will suffice to raise arterial PO_2 to an adequate level.

2   In pre-term infants, high concentrations of oxygen may cause *retrolental fibroplasia* of the eye, leading to blindness. In these patients arterial PO_2 should never be above 10 to 12 kPa (70 to 90 mmHg) depending on the gestational age.

4   Respiratory intensive care in particular conditions

The principles of respiratory intensive care, described so far, apply to a wide range of clinical conditions. The detailed management of many of these, e.g. tetanus, polyneuritis, chest injuries and overdosage with drugs, will not be further discussed. Three conditions, however, call for comment because they often complicate the management of other disorders.

Asthma

Asthma is characterized by the episodic occurrence of widespread obstruction affecting the small bronchi. The obstruction is due to muscular constriction, to oedema of the bronchial wall and to plugging of the lumen of the airway by sticky lumps of mucus. As the airways become more severely obstructed, hypoxia increases and eventually arterial PCO_2 begins to rise. The situation is then very serious and demands urgent treatment.

Treatment. Patients with asthma may be referred to an ICU early or late in the downhill course, and it is often difficult to decide how far the immediate treatment should go. This will not be discussed, but a brief statement is necessary of the various measures which may be required in these cases.

1　*Oxygen* is the first requirement, and may be given in high concentration by a suitable mask or, if intubation is needed, by ventilator. The aim is to keep arterial PO_2 above 13 kPa (100 mmHg) but even a high concentration of O_2 may not achieve this.

2　*Metabolic acidosis* is common in a prolonged attack, and impairs the action of bronchodilator and steroid drugs. If revealed by analysis of arterial blood, it must be corrected by the infusion of the proper amount of sodium bicarbonate.

3　*Hydration.* Patients with asthma are often dehydrated because they have been unable to take liquids and have breathed through their mouths for some time before admission to the ICU. Although it may seem logical to aid liquefaction of secretions by humidifying the inspired air this is difficult to accomplish and liquefaction of the secretions is best induced by rehydrating the patient with intravenous fluids.

4　*Bronchodilator drugs.* The patient entering an ICU will almost always have consumed, during the preceding hours or days, a large quantity of salbutamol, isoprenaline, orciprenaline or adrenaline (p. 33) by injection or aerosol, and will have become relatively or completely resistant to them. 'Resistance' may be due to the inability of aerosol to reach the small bronchi because of mucous plugging, but sometimes seems to be a true insensitivity to the drug. Sensitivity may be restored after acidosis has been corrected or by the administration of a large dose of steroid (see below). Bronchodilators are best given by aerosol inhalation from a ventilator with an efficient nebulizer; for an adult, 2 ml of 1 per cent isoprenaline or orciprenaline, or 1 ml of 0·5 per cent salbutamol, should be put in the nebulizer. Aminophylline (up to 0·5 g by slow intravenous injection) is often a very effective bronchodilator. It should be used with great caution in patients suffering from ischemic heart disease in whom sudden death (presumably from ventricular fibrillation) has been reported to occur following intravenous aminophylline.

5　*Steroids*, in big doses, often have a profound effect in asthma. How they work is conjectural, but it is well known that they modify allergic responses and that allergy plays an important part in the asthmatic attack. They also reduce bronchial oedema. An asthmatic patient who is ill enough to need intensive care almost always needs steroid treatment. Prednisone, 60 mg, or dexamethasone, 10 mg, should be given by mouth at once; dexamethasone or methylprednisolone may be given intravenously instead. High dosage must be continued for up to 5 days; thereafter, its advantages must be weighed against the risk of suppressing the patient's suprarenal glands.

6 *Antibiotics.* Pulmonary infection is so common in longstanding attacks of asthma that 'blind' antibiotic treatment is probably justifiable. The likely organisms are *Strept. penumoniae* and *H. influenzae*, and ampicillin is appropriate. Subsequent culture of sputum may prompt a change of antibiotic.

7 *Sedation*, especially in patients who are not being ventilated, must be given with great care, since the consequences of respiratory depression may be disastrous (p. 87). Diazepam is probably safe; paraldehyde is also acceptable but is disagreeable.

8 *Artificial ventilation* is usually required when arterial PO_2 is seriously depressed and arterial PCO_2 is rising (p. 246). The decision to ventilate is usually made, however, on clinical grounds, because the blood gases can deteriorate very quickly and acceptable levels provide little insurance against early disaster.

Severe asthma poses several problems in artificial ventilation:

a Unless the patient is heavily sedated or curarized he will 'fight the respirator', and manual ventilation by Ambu bag must often be given for long periods.

b Very high inflation pressures are needed, and these carry a serious risk of pneumothorax (p. 256).

c Lung compliance and airways resistance may change rapidly and asthmatic patients are thus best ventilated with a volume preset machine

d Expiration is greatly hampered by bronchoconstriction, and the expiratory phase has to be made to last longer than the usual two-thirds of the cycle (p. 252).

e Adequate intravenous hydration is vital, since secretions are thicker and stickier than in any other condition. The removal of mucous plugs is the principal concern of treatment at this stage. Instillation of isotonic saline solution, 'artificial coughing' and aspiration of the airway must be pursued patiently and continuously until improvement is well established. In some centres, bronchoscopic lavage is favoured. However it is difficult to maintain oxygenation during prolonged bronchoscopy and the place of this procedure is not finally established.

9 *Drugs to be avoided.* Morphine, papaveretum and other narcotics increase bronchoconstriction and should not be given even when the patient is being ventilated. Barbiturates, in doses adequate to sedate a patient with severe asthma, depress breathing and should not be used unless he is being artificially ventilated; even then, diazepam or promethazine is usually adequate. Finally, β-adrenergic blocking drugs such as propranolol are contraindicated in asthma because they are powerful brochoconstrictors.

Chronic bronchitis and emphysema

Patients with longstanding pulmonary damage due to bronchitis, bronchiectasis, dust diseases (pneumoconiosis,) tuberculosis (active and healed), chest deformity and other conditions form a group with similar problems which may call for intensive care. They all eventually die from ventilatory or cardiac failure, but these may be precipitated, usually by intercurrent respiratory infection, some years before the chronic disease has run its full course. When such a patient presents with ventilatory failure, a decision must be made as to whether this is mainly due to chronic, irreversible pulmonary damage or whether a reasonably good functional state has been severely impaired by an acute (and probably treatable) infection. This decision can be difficult to make.

The *management* of these patients follows the principles outlined on pp. 248 to 256.

Pneumothorax

When the pleural space on one or both sides of the chest contains air, a pneumothorax is present. The air may enter the pleural space from a leaking lung or bronchus, or it may be introduced through a hole in the chest wall (thoracotomy, pleural drain or trauma).

Air may escape from the lungs or bronchi under the following conditions.

1 When the lungs are apparently healthy, and for no obvious reason; this is the 'spontaneous pneumothorax' which is seen in relatively young people.

2 As a complication of emphysema or asthma, a distended air space may rupture through the pleura.

3 Acute pulmonary infection is sometimes complicated by pneumothorax.

4 In IPPV, particularly if inflation-pressure is high, a pneumothorax may occur. In this case the air usually escapes through the wall of a bronchus and tracks through the substance of the lung to the mediastinum, finally tearing the mediastinal pleura and entering the pleural space.

5 After injury, in which the lung may be torn by a broken rib (or during the insertion of a subclavian CVP line) or a bronchus may be ruptured by sudden stress on the thorax. Air may also leak from alveoli or from a bronchus following the resection of part of the lung.

Pressure in a pneumothorax. A pneumothorax may be small, with only partial collapse of the lung; in this case the pressure in the pneumothorax is still less than atmospheric. A bigger leak of air may cause complete collapse of the lung and the pneumothorax pressure may reach atmospheric. Sometimes, especially when respiratory obstruction is present, air continues to enter the pleural space until its pressure is considerably greater than atmospheric; this is called a *tension pneumothorax*. When this happens, the heart and other mediastinal structures are pushed towards the opposite side of the chest, and serious circulatory and respiratory embarrassment may arise very quickly. Pneumothorax, especially tension pneumothorax, is sometimes accompanied by 'surgical emphysema' — air under the skin of the chest wall, head and neck.

The *diagnosis* of pneumothorax can often be made with certainty on clinical grounds. A chest x-ray resolves all doubt.

Treatment. A small pneumothorax which is not getting bigger can usually be left alone and will be absorbed spontaneously. A bigger one or one which is increasing in size, or a pneumothorax which is interfering with ventilation or circulation, demands the insertion of one or more intercostal drainage tubes. These are connected to an underwater seal which is placed well below the level of the patient's chest. The principle of underwater drainage is illustrated in Fig. 52

(p. 177) but, for pleural drains, suction is not always used and the short tube is left open. The underwater seal acts as a one-way valve allowing air to escape from the chest without allowing the entry of air through the tube. The vessel and the tubing should be made of clear material so that the fluid levels can be observed. During inspiration the negative intrathoracic pressure sucks some of the fluid upwards into the underwater tube while expiration lowers the level because of the relative increase in intrathoracic pressure. This fluctuation of fluid in the underwater tube is normal.

Air present in the pleural space will bubble from the underwater seal during expiration and this is increased by deep expiratory effort or coughing. Once the lung is completely expanded, the underwater seal stops bubbling and fluctuation in the underwater tube stops because the re-expanded lung blocks the openings of the drain into the pleural space. The intercostal drainage tube is removed when a chest x-ray has confirmed re-expansion of the lung.

An underwater drain that continues to bubble indicates a continuous leak of air into the pleural cavity. Under these circumstances great care should be taken that the underwater drain is not blocked in any way as the pneumothorax would immediately recur and a tension pneumothorax may develop. Occasionally the air leak is so great that the lung does not re-expand when an intercostal drain is inserted. When this occurs, gentle suction (0·5 to 2·5 kPa or 5 to 20 mmHg) is applied to the short tube of the underwater seal so that air may be removed faster than it accumulates in the pleural cavity. The use of suction often decreases fluctuation of the fluid in the underwater tube. If the suction system fails for any reason it must immediately be disconnected from the underwater seal or it will block the escape of air.

Sometimes the use of suction prevents the natural sealing of a leak and perpetuates the pneumothorax. In such cases active suction may have to be stopped but, if the pneumothorax recurs, surgical closure of the leak may be indicated.

Tension pneumothorax calls for urgent relief by the insertion or replacement of intercostal tubes. At times a wide needle, plunged through the chest wall, may be life-saving; air can be heard to hiss from the needle as the big pneumothorax is deflated.

When respiratory obstruction is present, surgical emphysema may persist and even increase despite apparently adequate deflation of the pneumothorax. This is because the cutaneous emphysema does not arise from the pneumothorax itself, but from the bronchial leak which gives rise to both. Tracheal intubation or tracheostomy may be neccessary to relieve the respiratory obstruction and thus the high intrabronchial pressure which is present during straining, coughing and even ordinary breathing.

Partial and total lung resection. After partial resection of the lung (*lobectomy*) the space in the pleural cavity is filled mainly by expansion of the portion of lung remaining. Intercostal drainage tubes are used to remove air, blood and serum from the pleural cavity so that the re-expansion of the lung is not hindered. These intercostal drains are managed in the same way as a drain placed for a pneumothorax.

After total resection of one lung (*pneumonectomy*) there is no lung left to fill the pleural cavity, and the space has to be filled with blood, blood clot, fluid and air. It is obvious therefore that the intercostal drain should remain clamped after pneumonectomy. If this space is accidentally drained, the heart and other mediastinal structures move across to fill it causing serious circulatory embarrassment. The only reason that an intercostal tube is left in position after pneumonectomy is so that it can be used to adjust the position of the mediastinum by allowing controlled amounts of air to enter, or escape from, the pleural space while monitoring the position of the mediastinum on chest x-ray.

12 Care of Infants and Small Children

To simplify the account in previous sections, treatment has generally been described for adult patients. While the essentials of treatment in infants and children are the same as in adults, there are many major practical differences. The infant is by no means merely a small edition of an adult, and the nursing of sick infants requires special experience, skill and care. An adult can adjust to quite big changes in his environment and can compensate, to some extent, for surgical complications or minor errors in management. The very young child lacks this capacity and treatment of the infant must therefore be very precise.

At first, attempts at surgical correction of cardiac defects in infants were associated with a high mortality. The main problems lay in the access inside tiny hearts with cannulae in place for cardiopulmonary bypass, and in the much smaller perfusion rates and priming volumes required compared with adults. In recent years, technical improvements have reduced the risks of cardiopulmonary bypass, and the use of profound hypothermia has further extended the scope of surgery. In the latter technique, the infant is cooled to about 18°C, either by surface cooling with ice bags or by perfusion with cold blood from a heart-lung machine. Blood is then drained into the machine and the cardiac defect corrected in a relaxed and bloodless heart. Circulatory arrest is well tolerated for 1 hr at this temperature. Rewarming is generally carried out by perfusion with warm blood.

Many anomalies can now be corrected in infancy. The postoperative care differs little whether correction has been carried out during cardiopulmonary bypass or under profound hypothermia and circulatory arrest. In general, the more complex the initial cardiac defect, the more demanding is postoperative management.

Special problems in the first week of life

The birth of an infant is the most severe test of physiological adaptation he will face in his life time. Detailed consideration of the changes which occur before and after birth is beyond the scope of this book, and the ICU nurse would do well to refer to a text of neonatal care. Fortunately, infants have usually overcome the immediate problems associated with delivery and adaptation to extrauterine life by the time they need treatment of cardiac disease. Even so, the young infant's response to stress differs in many ways from that of the older infant, and it is imperative that this be recognized in management. Difficulties are specially likely in the *premature infant* (gestational age less than 37 weeks) and in the *low-birth weight* infant (weight less than 2·5 kg). With premature infants there is an increased incidence of idiopathic respiratory distress of the newborn, intracranial haemorrhage, apnoeic attacks, problems with temperature control, jaundice, infections, and feeding problems. With low-birth weight infants who are small for dates there is an increased incidence of hypoxia and cerebral trauma at birth, meconium aspiration, pulmonary haemorrhage, problems with temperature control, hypoglycaemia and polycythemia.

Circulatory system

The circulation of a newborn infant demands particular attention. The pulmonary resistance-vessels are very muscular at birth and if the infant becomes hypoxic or acidotic these vessels constrict strongly, producing a sharp rise in pulmonary vascular resistance. Perfusion of the lungs is impaired, hypoxia becomes more marked, and a vicious cycle is set up, leading rapidly to a fall in cardiac output. During the first few days a right-to-left shunt occurs readily through the foramen ovale or the still-patent ductus arteriosus, resulting in further reduction in pulmonary blood-flow and increasing systemic hypoxia. This situation is described as the *transitional circulation*. Attention is paid to any stressful influence, e.g. hypothermia or infection; acidosis is treated with bicarbonate administration, IPPV is administered if necessary to provide adequate ventilation (the primary indication being a high PCO_2) and if necessary a pulmonary vasodilator is added. There is no perfect pulomonary vasodilator, all available agents having the disadvantage that they also dilate systemic vessels, and having individual side effects. The greatest experience in the newborn period is probably with tolazaline, given intravenously at a dosage of 1 to 2 mg per kg over 10 min and 1 to 2 mg per kg hourly thereafter. In the normal infant the thickness and reactivity of the pulmonary vessels diminish from birth to reach a stable level by 2 or 3 weeks of age. In infants with cardiac disease, however, the vessels may remain hyperreactive for months.

Respiratory system

At birth the infant must transform unaerated, fluid-filled lungs to aerated, expanded structures capable of supporting respiration. Not surprisingly problems with this dramatic transformation are common, particularly in premature and small for dates babies. The most common problem is idiopathic respiratory distress of the newborn (IRDS). IRDS is due mainly to inadequate production of surfactant and is most common in premature infants. Treatment includes adequate oxygenation and ventilatory assistance with a distending pressure, either CPAP or, in the more severe cases, IPPV usually with PEEP (p. 257) Optimal fluid balance is important.

Two conditions may present in the ICU at this time. One of these is *tracheo-oesophageal fistula*. In its commonest form, there is an interruption of the oesophagus, the lower part of which has a fistulous connection with the trachea (Fig. 75). Other anatomical variants occur. Diagnosis at birth is essential, or severe respiratory problems arise from aspiration from the upper pouch or fistula. The condition may be suspected when a firm 10 to 13 French tube cannot be passed beyond 9 to 13 cm from the nares, and may be confirmed by instilling a little contrast material into the oesophagus and taking an x-ray film. The fistula must be surgically divided and, when possible, the ends of the oesophagus joined; usually a gastrostomy is made. Chest drains are kept in place until drainage is minimal. When gastric function returns, intravenous fluids are replaced by small gastrostomy feeds. Some days later, another x-ray will confirm that the oesophageal anastomosis is satisfactory and oral feeding is then begun.

Diaphragmatic hernia also calls for immediate surgical treatment. In this condition the abdominal contents protrude into the chest

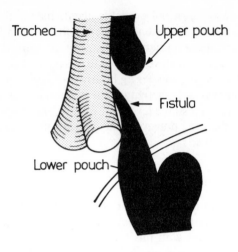

Fig. 75 The most common anatomy in oesophageal atresia, present in over 80 per cent of cases. More rarely either the atresia or the fistula may occur alone, or an upper fistula or double fistula may be present.

through a defect in the diaphragm, producing severe compression of the lungs. The defect can be corrected surgically, but one or both lungs may have failed to develop owing to prolonged compression *in utero*. In this case severe hypoventilation and hypoxia may persist despite operation, and some infants have so little functioning lung that survival is impossible. Postoperative management includes maintenance of IPPV and, where intense pulmonary vasoconstriction is a major feature, administration of a pulmonary vasodilator. Over the first few hours it usually becomes apparent whether or not there is any chance of survival.

Temperature control

Because they have a relatively high surface area and modest stores of subcutaneous fat, infants are more vulnerable to heat loss than are older patients and also less able to generate heat. When exposed to cold an adult increases heat production by voluntary muscle activity, involuntary muscle activity (shivering) and by 'non-shiving thermogenesis'. Only the third mechanism is well developed in the newborn, so that mobilising fatty acids from brown fat stores is the main method of thermal control. A normal infant may increase metabolic activity almost threefold in an attempt to maintain body temperature (Fig. 76). Recognition of this mechanism is vital in the management of an infant with a critically low cardiac output — exposing the baby to cold may be the last straw. It is important also to realise that a normal rectal temperature does not guarantee that the baby's ambient temperature is ideal as he may be maintaining a normal rectal temperature only by intense metabolic activity. The *neutral thermal environmental temperature* at which metabolic activity is minimal depends on gestational and chronological age, and weight. Examples are shown in Table 16. For most infants the range is 32 to 34°C, but for young, small infants it may be up to 35°C (Fig. 76). If an infant is nursed in an incubator, heat loss may occur by radiation and this can be minimised by covering him with a diaper. Nursing under a radiant heater is now generally preferred but this does not exclude lateral radiation. Whichever method is used it is important that the ICU shall be warm and

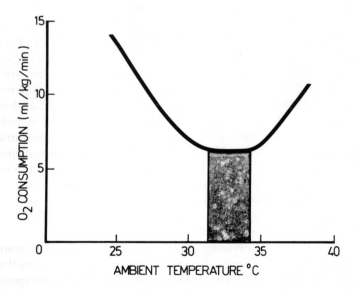

Fig. 76 Relation between ambient temperature and metabolic activity in infancy.

Table 16 Neutral thermal environment temperature of the newborn.

Age	Weight (g)		Range of temperature °C)
First 2 days	< 1200		34–35
	> 2500	(> 36 weeks	32–34
5–6	< 1500	gestational age)	31–32
	1500–2500		29–32

draught-free. Approximately 1°C must be added to the ambient temperature of a child in an incubator for every 7°C difference between room and incubator temperature. Abdominal cutaneous temperature should be monitored and kept as close as possible to 36·2°C in a full-term infant and 36·5°C in a small for dates infant. Rectal temperature should not differ by more than 1·5°C from abdominal cutaneous temperature. After heart surgery an infant often becomes pyrexial. This produces a similar increase in metabolic activity, and should be controlled as well as possible.

Resistance to infection is limited in the newborn and does not approach adult efficiency for many months. Humoral defences are relatively weak. IgG antibodies, important in resisting streptococcal and haemophilus infections, have crossed the placenta but levels fall over the first 3 to 5 months. IgM antibodies, important for Gram negative infections, and IgA antibodies, important for gastrointestinal infections, build up only slowly from birth. Cell-mediated phagocytosis (lymphocytes), important for viral and fungal infections, is deficient. Humoral-mediated phagocytosis (neutrophils) is also weak, the initial action of plasma proteins and complement being limited.

The young infant is very susceptible to infection and symptoms and signs tend to be poorly localised. Meningitis and septicaemia in particular may cause few of the classical signs; the baby is just unresponsive and unwell. Pneumonia also may be relatively 'silent'. In such cases other evidence (chest x-ray, lumbar puncture, blood culture, etc.) are required for diagnosis and antibiotics are given while awaiting results. This tendency to 'atypical' presentation of infection persists for many months and must therefore be borne in mind with all infants undergoing cardiac operations.

Nutrition and metabolism

A newborn will usually take only about 75 calories per kg per day but by 1 week a full-term infant requires 100 calories per kg per day. Human milk, and most milk formulae in usual dilution, contain about 67 calories per 100 ml, so that fluid intake is about 130 ml per kg per day. Under ideal conditions a premature infant may be able to utilise 40 per cent of his caloric intake for growth, but to achieve this he may need 150 calories per kg per day. Because of limitations in handling fluid load and the limited caloric content of infused fluids, these conditions are not approached in the first days after cardiac surgery. Although the inadequate caloric intake is tolerated for 2 to 3 days, it becomes a major problem if prolonged.

Some enzyme systems are relatively underdeveloped in the newborn, especially in the premature infant. For example the limitation of uptake and conjugation of bilirubin by liver cells is a major reason for the frequency with which *jaundice* is seen in the newborn period. Apart from well-recognized causes ('physiological' jaundice, haemolytic disease etc.) it is seen with many infections and even with haematomata and bruising. Chronic liver congestion will prolong the jaundice.

This serves as a reminder of the need for great care in the administration of drugs, many of which are metabolised in the liver. *Hypoglycaemia* occurs readily in the newborn, especially at times of stress and undernutrition. Pallor, failure to feed, limpness or unresponsiveness may be the only signs of a blood glucose concentration below 1·7 mmol per l (30 mg per 100 ml), which can cause serious brain damage unless treated promptly. An IV infusion of glucose is needed, sometimes about 3 ml per kg per hr of 10 to 15 per cent glucose. Hypoglycaemic convulsions are a late sign, and may amount to no more than mild twitching of one limb. *Hypocalcaemia* is another cause of convulsive twitching. *Any abnormal movements, however slight, may indicate the presence of a serious and treatable infection or metabolic abnormality, and must be investigated at once.*

Drugs in infancy and childhood

Excretion of drugs by the kidneys and their metabolism by the liver are functions which are incompletely developed in the newborn. Side effects, therefore, occur more readily and tend to be more severe than in older patients. On the other hand, infants and small children, weight for weight, are metabolically more active than adults, and per kg of weight they need relatively bigger doses of drugs. Thus a newborn baby weighs only one-twentieth as much as an adult, but usually needs one-tenth of an adult's daily dose of a drug. At 1 year the daily dose is approximately one-quarter, at 3 years one-third, and at 7 years, one-half of an adult's. There are, however, many exceptions to this rule. Table 17 (p. 285) shows the dosage for infants of some commonly used drugs. Premature and low-birth weight babies should receive the lower dose in each case. Morphine, vitamin K, chloramphenicol and sulphonamides may cause disastrous side effects unless given with great care.

Prolonged infusion of drugs in infants and small children may make fluid balance difficult to manage. The simplest method is to give each drug in relatively concentrated solutions from a constant-infusion pump, by means of which a very slow infusion may be given with great accuracy, and the rate changed at will without encroaching too much upon the water requirement. Needless to say, the volume delivered, though small, must be reckoned in the 24 hr balance chart. Whether pumps are used or not, it is good practice to separate the drips by which different drugs, electrolytes and nutrients are being given, so that dosages can be varied singly as far as necessary.

Postoperative care of infants following cardiac surgery

The infant's environment

The infant is nursed under a radiant heater in a warm, draught-free ICU. A cutaneous temperature of $36 \cdot 2°$ to $36 \cdot 5°C$ is aimed at, usually requiring an ambient temperature of $32°$ to $34°C$. If pyrexia occurs, ambient temperature is reduced, aspirin or paracetamol may be administered and tepid sponging may be used.

The baby is washed daily with soap and water. In young infants the cord is swabbed at each feeding time with iodophor in alcohol. Oral thrush, due to infection with a yeast *Candida albicans*, is common; this is treated with mycostatin (1 ml of a solution containing 100 000 units per ml) after each feed or 4-hourly with a $0 \cdot 75$ per cent gentian violet solution. Other infections are dealt with appropriately (p. 124).

It must be emphasised that the most important part of treatment is *prevention of infection*. All equipment must be cleaned regularly according to a strict routine and barrier nursing must be meticulously maintained. If incubators are used they should be changed every 48 hr, their exteriors dampdusted daily and their interiors kept free from condensation.

Water, electrolytes and nutrition

Fluid intake is strictly limited for the first 48 hr after operation, the infant usually receiving only 2 ml of 5 per cent glucose solution per kg per hr intravenously. Salt and water are retained avidly (pp. 24–183). The presence of oedema, often first noticed as puffiness of the eyelids, indicates fluid overload. A low serum sodium almost always indicates water overload, not sodium depletion; this is true especially if oedema is present. Water requirement is reduced if the baby is breathing humidified air or oxygen, as significant volumes of water can be absorbed from the lungs. Requirements tend to be higher in infants nursed under a radiant heat warmer and intake is, of course, increased if losses occur from the gastrointestinal tract or other drainage. The solution used to flush pressure-lines must be reckoned as part of the intake and recorded carefully. Infusion cannulae must be protected and handled aseptically, the infusion-set changed daily and the limb watched carefully for leakage from, or thrombosis of the vein.

Potassium chloride must usually be added to the infusion at a rate of 1 to 2 mmol per kg per day, but more may be added during the first 8 hr when, if all is going well, the serum potassium concentration tends to fall. Little or no sodium is needed at first, but after 48 hr the usual requirement is about 2 mmol per kg per day. The recommended infusion rate provides only 2·5 g of glucose per kg per day, equivalent to 10 Cal (42 kJ) per kg per day, barely one quarter of the amount required to minimise protein breakdown. Such a negative metabolic balance is acceptable for a short time, but it is essential to increase the intake as soon as possible. Regular estimations of blood glucose concentration are needed during the first few days to detect any tendency to hypoglycaemia.

Oral feeding is deferred for at least 24 hr after operation because of the risk of regurgitation and inhalation of gastric contents. A start may be made with 5 to 10 ml of 5 per cent glucose solution 2-hourly;

it should be recognised that this is probably as irritant, if inhaled, as milk, but at least it does not form curds. If the first glucose feeds are taken well, milk may be introduced; either breast milk or an adapted milk formula (e.g. 'Enfamil' or 'SMA') given undiluted. It is wise to continue frequent feeds for up to 48 hr but, if small feeds are well tolerated, their volume is rapidly increased, the rate of intravenous infusion being correspondingly tapered off.

A baby too weak or too breathless to suck has to be fed by nasogastric tube, which is usually best left in position between feeds. The total distance from the bridge of the baby's nose to the ear, and from ear to xiphisternum, is measured, and this length of tube is inserted. Before each feed, the position of the tube should be checked by aspirating the stomach contents (recording the volume aspirated) and confirming that they are acid to litmus; the acid content of gastric juice in the premature infant is, however, sometimes low. In *sick babies. the volume of fluid given by nasogastric feeding is the same as would be given by the intravenous route.*

If a baby inhales gastric contents an endotracheal tube must be passed so that the bronchi may be aspirated. Ventilation can then be assisted through the endotracheal tube. A gastric tube, if not already in place, should be passed and the stomach emptied. Throughout, a watch must be kept for cardiac arrest and cardiac massage given if necessary. A steroid drug is often given in an attempt to minimise the chemical pneumonia due to inhaled gastric acid, and an antibiotic is necessary.

Where nasogastric feed is inadvisable, IV alimentation must be considered.

Maintenance of cardiac output

Assuming that the basic requirements of temperature control, oxygenation, and water, electrolytes and nutrition are met, the greatest postoperative problems are low cardiac output and respiratory difficulties. Either of these can cause sudden disaster, and the utmost vigilence is needed to detect their earliest signs.

Diagnosis of low cardiac output

1 Ideally, cardiac output should be measured regularly during the first 48 hr following operation, but this is often difficult.

2 A cool periphery despite an adequate core temperature is an indication of low output.

3 Decline in urinary output: despite the risk of infection, catheterisation of the bladder is essential if there is any doubt about cardiac output. A urinary volume of 1 ml per kg per hr is satisfactory; a fall to less than 0·5 ml is ominous.

4 An increasing serum potassium concentration (except for that induced by potassium supplements) has a similar significance. Progressive change is the most important sign but a level exceeding 5 mmol per l from a venous sample demands attention.

5 An increasing base deficit (p. 16) usually indicates inadequate tissue perfusion, although it is also a feature of sustained hypoxia. Progressive changes are more significant than a single value, but the situation should be reviewed if the base deficit exceeds 5 to 6 mmol per l.

6 Intense peripheral vasoconstriction and a fall in arterial pressure are late signs of a reduced cardiac output, and infants may die before these become obvious.

7 To detect the first signs, measurements of base deficit and serum potassium are required 2-hourly, and sometimes more often, in the initial stages. Low arterial Po_2 and high Pco_2 add urgency.

Treatment. Provided the signs of a low cardiac output are recognised early enough, prompt treatment will usually carry the infant through the critical period. Tamponade (p. 189) and blood loss (p. 188) whould be excluded or treated. In their absence the following measures may be taken:

1 Satisfactory filling pressures are ensured, bearing in mind the underlying cardiac problem. Pressures of 10 to 12 mmHg are usually optimal.

2 Rapid digitalisation, provided that serum potassium has stabilized.

3 Infusion of isoprenaline (0·1 to 0·5 μg per kg per min), dopamine or dobutamine (2·5 to 10 μg per kg per min).

4 Cardiac pacing, preferably atrial, to maintain the heart rate at about 120 per min.

5 Intravenous frusemide (1 to 2 mg per kg) to increase urinary output.

6 Intravenous sodium bicarbonate to correct any base deficit.

7 Ventilatory support to correct hypoxia and hypercapnia. If Pco_2

is satisfactory, CPAP may be sufficient but IPPV, in addition to improving $P\text{CO}_2$, removes the work of ventilation.

8 Use of a vasodilator, most commonly sodium nitroprusside at a dosage of 0·5 to 4 μg per kg per min.

9 If serum potassium rises above 6 mmol per l in a venous sample, 1 to 2 units of insulin covered by 2 g of glucose per unit may be required. If urinary output does not increase with the above measures and potassium continues to rise, peritoneal dialysis must be considered. Equipment for dialysis suitable for use in infants is kept in readiness in the ICU.

It is often necessary to continue treatment for up to 48 hr, and sometimes for several days.

Respiration

The maintenance of optimal arterial blood $P\text{O}_2$ demands reliable control of the oxygen concentration of the inspired gas. Oxygen is usually administered through a plastic head box and the concentration is checked frequently. The required concentration is usually dictated by the infant's condition, but with high concentrations the risk of pulmonary oxygen toxicity should be remembered (p. 261). Premature infants, especially those of less than 34 weeks' gestation, may develop retrolental fibroplasia if arterial $P\text{O}_2$ is kept at an abnormally high level, and this can occur with ambient oxygen levels as low as 40 per cent over several hours. Continuous monitoring with a transcutaneous $P\text{O}_2$ monitor with periodic checks of arterial $P\text{O}_2$ protect against this.

Respiratory effort and the force of coughing are weaker in the newborn and young infant, and secretions readily accumulate causing patchy collapse of the lungs. For a time the infant will cope with the increased work of breathing (p. 71) but soon becomes exhausted and slips into ventilatory failure (pp. 87, 248) with hypoxia and even cardiac arrest. Even a small haemothorax or pneumothorax may have a similar result.

The infant's breathing must therefore be observed carefully. Although the normal respiratory frequency varies widely from one infant to another (30 to 50 per min), an *increasing* frequency is often an early sign of respiratory distress. At other times unusually slow, laboured breathing indicates imminent disaster. With pulmonary collapse, obstruction of the airways or pulmonary congestion, indrawing of the lower ribs or suprasternal tissues will often be seen. Should these signs develop, the pharynx (and bronchial tree if the baby is intubated) should be aspirated and further steps set in train. An infant may need urgent intubation and equipment for this must be immediately at hand. Haemothorax, pneumothorax and atelectasis may be detected or confirmed by x-ray.

The arterial Po_2 and Pco_2 need to be measured frequently and allow accurate assessment of the respiratory state and the need for tracheal intubation. If the blood gases indicate the necessity for respiratory support, either CPAP or IPPV is begun. IPPV (p. 250) is usually required if the Pco_2 is more than 6·5 kPa (50 mmHg); CPAP (p. 257) is preferred if the Pco_2 is normal but the Po_2 is low.

In infants CPAP applied through an endotracheal tube is often used prophylactically during the first postoperative day or two,

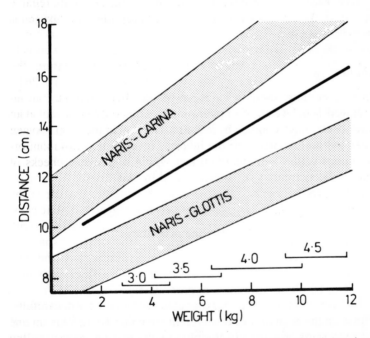

Fig. 77 Graph showing length and size (internal diameter in mm) of nasotracheal tubes related to weight. Shaded areas show 95 per cent limits of naris-carina and naris-glottis distances. Line between shaded areas shows naris-mid trachea distance; figures below show tube size.

since this technique, in addition to preventing atelectasis, allows:
(a) aspiration of secretions,
(b) accurate delivery of a known concentration of oxygen and
(c) manual ventilation of the lungs, if indicated.
CPAP is also useful when a baby is being 'weaned' from IPPV.

An uncuffed tube is used, the size permitting a leak at 20 to 25 cm H_2O (Fig. 77). Fixing of the tracheal tube is difficult in infants. Undue movement of a nasotracheal tube will damage the trachea, larynx and nose, and the nurse must always take the greatest care to prevent this. She should obtain assistance when aspirating the trachea and when turning a baby to ensure that the various attachments are not twisted or pulled upon. The infant is very sensitive to periods of apnoea. The endotracheal tube has a seal through which a suction tube can be passed. This allows suctioning without interruption of ventilation.

Dry gases are harmful to the lungs and humidification is required. Where sticky secretions are a problem an ultrasonic nebuliser is used.

Fat necrosis

Surface cooling, used to induce profound hypothermia, may be followed 1 to 2 weeks after operation by fat necrosis in areas which have been directly cooled by ice bags. The subcutaneous tissues are inflamed and painful, and the infant is feverish and irritable. The condition settles without treatment within a couple of weeks. If necessary, symptoms can be alleviated by small doses of corticosteroid drugs.

Other routine procedures

Blood replacement

An infant's blood volume is approximately 75 to 85 ml per kg. Blood loss greater than 10 per cent of blood volume normally merits replacement in an infant. In an infant weighing 10 kg a loss of 200 ml represents a quarter of the blood volume. Special care is thus needed to note and measure blood loss and replace it; this includes blood taken for laboratory tests. Should more than one third of the blood volume be lost (or less, if loss is rapid) exploration of the wound in the operating theatre is usually called for. The loss of clotting factors (p. 188) should be kept in mind whenever substantial blood replacement is necessary. The newborn infant may be deficient in clotting factors even before bleeding has occurred, and quickly becomes more depleted. It is usual to give vitamin K in the delivery suite; if bleeding occurs later, a further dose (1 mg intramuscularly) may be needed, and other clotting factors supplied by infusing freeze-dried plasma or fresh blood. Because a blood prime is used for bypass, the haemoglobin may be relatively high in the initial postoperative period. In this case plasma rather than whole blood may be used for volume replacement.

Postoperative pain

Pain can be relieved with morphine or papaveretum in repeated, small intravenous doses, usually about 0·1 mg per kg per dose. Provided a cause requiring specific treatment can be excluded, restlessness may be relieved with small intravenous doses of diazepam, usually about 0·1 to 0·2 mg per kg. The infant should lie comfortably with nothing pressing on his wound or pulling on drainage or nasogastric tubes. A dummy is often a comfort to him and for the older child the favourite teddy bear may be an invaluable bedfellow, even if it fails to satisfy the rules of sterility in every respect. The need to minimise mental stress in children in the ICU will need no emphasis to a good nurse.

Prostaglandin administration

Some infants, for example those with pulmonary atresia, depend on patency of the ductus arteriosus for survival. In the first weeks of life the ductus can be kept open with an infusion of prostaglandin E1. The full dosage is about 0·1 μg per kg per min but it is usual to start an infusion, when the infant shows progressive hypoxia, with about one quarter of this dosage. Hypotension and apnoea can occur at the onset of treatment so that arterial pressures must be monitored and facilities for ventilation must be at hand. Where palliative surgery is planned it is usual to continue the infusion of PGE1 until the operation is under way. Prostaglandins are also useful in a number of other conditions. In an infant with interruption of the aorta or extreme coarctation, critical deterioration may occur as the ductus closes. The situation can be temporarily reversed by reopening the ductus.

Infants with Ebstein's anomaly may develop gross hypoxia in the neonatal period, due to the leak of the tricuspid valve and consequent right to left shunt at atrial level. As pulmonary arteriolar resistance gradually falls after birth, the baby's condition may improve. PGE1 may allow survival by maintaining pulmonary flow through the patent ductus while this process occurs, the additional pulmonary vasodilator action of PGE1 helping the process along. This pulmonary vasodilator action also appears helpful in those few infants with simple transposition of the great arteries who remain severely hypoxic after balloon septostomy. Maintenance of patency of the ductus arteriosus and reduction of pulmonary vascular resistance probably both help, the first by directly increasing the shunt from aorta to pulmonary artery and the second by increasing blood flow and creating turbulence in the atria, probably allowing better mixing at that level.

Psychosocial considerations

All nurses recognise the need to protect the baby as far as possible from fear and pain, and to soothe and comfort him. Equally important is support of his parents, for whom the postoperative period is tense and frightening. They are prepared as well as possible by a preoperative visit to the ICU and by discussions and illustrations showing drainage tubes and equipment. They are encouraged to be present as much as they wish in the ICU, and to handle their baby, even if this only means holding his hand in the first day or so. As soon as possible they should be able to cuddle him and help with his feeding. If the operation comes very early in the baby's life, separation can seriously interfere with mothering and, if later, the parents feel very helpless in the ICU situation. Understanding and firmness are both required, as the infant must not be deprived of necessary treatment because of parental anxiety. Parents can usually accept the need for therapeutic procedures if these are adequately explained. Support of relatives is further discussed (pp. 187, 214 and 236).

Table 17 Dosage levels for infants of some commonly used drugs.

Drug	Parenteral dose unless otherwise stated (oral doses are usually somewhat higher)
Antibiotics	
Amikacin	Loading: 10 mg per kg followed by 7·5 mg per kg every 12 hours
Amoxycillin	125 mg three times daily (oral)
Ampicillin	100–400 mg per kg per day
Benzathine penicillin	300 000 units – 600 000 units/single dose
Benzylpenicillin	30–150 mg per kg per day (50 000–250 000 units)
Carbenicillin	100–500 mg per kg per day
Cefoxitin	100 mg per kg per day
Cephalexin	50–100 mg per kg per day (oral)
Cephradine	50–100 mg per kg per day (oral or injection)
Cloxacillin	50–100 mg per kg per day
Erythromycin	12 mg per kg per day
Flucloxacillin	125 mg three times daily (oral)
Gentamicin	5–7·5 mg per kg per day
Ticarcillin	Newborn 100 mg per kg 1st dose, then 300–450 mg per kg per day. Over 2 weeks of age, 600 mg per kg per day
Tobramycin	3–7·5 mg per kg per day
Cardiac drugs	
Adrenaline	2 μg per kg emergency dose. Otherwise for isoprenaline.
Alprostadil (Prostaglandin E1)	0·025–0·1 μg/kg/minute
Digoxin	**a** *Total digitalizing dose (given over 24 hours)* Premature babies: 0·05 mg per kg. (50 μg per kg) Infants: 0·05 to 0·07 mg per kg (50–70 μg per kg) Over 2 years 0·05 mg per kg. (50 μg per kg) **b** *Daily Maintenance* Premature babies 0·01 mg per kg (10 μg per kg) Infants: 0·01–0·02 mg per kg (10–20 μg per kg) Over 2 years: 0·01–0·015 mg per kg (10–15 μg per kg)

Table 17 continued overleaf

Table 17 continued

Drug	Parenteral dose unless otherwise stated (oral doses are usually somewhat higher)
Cardiac drugs Digoxin (cont.)	Digitalizing dose is given orally or intramuscularly. Maintenance doses are usually given orally. Intramuscular maintenance dose is about $\frac{2}{3}$ of the oral dose. Toxic levels still occur on these doses especially in premature infants and those with low cardiac output
Disopyramide	2 mg per kg in 1 hr; thereafter 0·4 mg per kg per hr
Dopamine	2·5–5 μg (rarely 10 μg) per kg per minute
Heparin	1 mg (100 units) per kg 4-hourly
Isoprenaline	0·5 μg per kg per min (maximal dose)
Lignocaine	0·5 to 1·0 mg per kg IV in 30 sec 0·03 to 0·1 mg per kg per min maintenance
Proscillaridin	Loading dose: 100 μg per kg in first 24 hr (oral) Maintenance: 25 μg per kg per day (oral)
Sodium nitroprusside	0·5–4 μg per kg per min
Tolazoline	1–2 mg per kg in 10 min, then 1–2 mg per kg per hr
Diuretics Amiloride	0·5–0·75 mg per kg per day (oral)
Chlorothiazide	30–50 mg per kg per day (oral)
Frusemide	1–2 mg per kg per day
Spironolactone	3 mg per kg per day
Steroids Dexamethasone	1–2 mg per kg initial dose 0·25 mg per kg per day maintenance
Anticonvulsants Paraldehyde	0·25 ml per kg dose
Phenobarbitone	3–10 mg per kg dose
Phenytoin sodium	4 mg per kg initial dose; 3–8 mg per kg per day maintenance
Sedatives (oral doses) Diazepam	0·2 mg per kg per dose (older children only)
Phenobarbitone	0·5–3 mg per kg per dose
Trimeprazine	1–4 mg per kg per dose

Table 17 continued

Drug	Parenteral dose unless otherwise stated (oral doses are usually somewhat higher)
Analgesics	
Aspirin	30–60 mg per kg per day (given with extreme care in infants)
Morphine hydrochloride	0·05–0·2 mg per kg per dose
Papaveretum	0·1–0·2 mg per kg per dose
Antagonist	
Naloxone (IV)	10 μg per kg (repeated at 2–3 min intervals if necessary)

IV Appendices, Recommended Reading and Index

Appendix 1
The Emergency Trolley

The trolley carries a portable oxygen cylinder, a portable suction pump, a defibrillator with appropriate leads and conducting paste and an 'Anglepoise' type lamp.

Drawer 1

Intravenous equipment, solutions and drugs

Intravenous catheters, assorted sizes
Tourniquet
2 filtered blood transfusion sets
2 infusion sets each with 100 ml graduated chamber
Dual injection site
Syringes, assorted sizes
200 ml molar sodium bicarbonate solution
500 ml 4·2 per cent dextrose in one-fifth isotonic saline
500 ml 5 per cent dextrose
500 ml stable plasma protein solution
Ampoule files
Lignocaine 2 per cent
Calcium chloride 1 mmol/ml
Adrenaline 1/10 000
Isoprenaline 1/5000
Dexamethasone 8 mg in 2 ml
Atropine 0·6 mg in 1 ml

Drawer 2

Adult intubation equipment

Oral suction
Oral airways: sizes 1, 2, 3

2 adult-size anaesthetic masks
1 Ambu bag
2 laryngoscopes
Disposable cuffed endotracheal tubes: sizes 6, 7, 8 and 9 mm
Malleable endotracheal tube introducer
Lignocaine jelly (2 per cent) for lubricating endotracheal tube
Magill laryngeal forceps
1 plastic 20 ml syringe for inflation of cuff
1 pair artery forceps with covered blades
1 catheter mount
Sterile suction catheters FG 12, 14, 16
Y piece to fit suction catheters
Gauze bandage and adhesive plaster

Drawer 3

Infant intubation equipment

Oral suction
3 infant-size oral airways
3 infant-size anaesthetic masks
Infant Ambu bag
2 largyngoscopes with small curved and straight blades
Disposable uncuffed endotracheal tubes: sizes 2·5, 3, 4 and 5 mm
Malleable endotracheal tube introducer
Lignocaine jelly (2 per cent) for lubricating endotracheal tube
Infant Magill laryngeal forceps
1 catheter mount
Sterile suction catheters FG 6, 8, 10
Y piece to fit suction catheters
Jackson-Rees infant T-piece and bag
Gauze bandage and adhesive plaster

The emergency trolley is checked daily and after use.

Appendix 2   Commonly Used Drugs

Table 18   Routes of administration: O, orally; Inj, by injection, either intravenous or intramuscular; IV, intravenous only; IM, intramuscular only; Inhal, by inhalation; R, rectally; Local app, local application.

Approved name		Commonly proprietary names	Route	Usual adult dose
British	American			
Acebutalol	Acebutalol	Sectral	IV	25 mg dose
			O	200–400 mg daily
Adrenaline	Epinephrine	Adrenaline (US)	IV	100–250 μg
(as acid tartrate)			SC	100–500 μg
Alprenolol		—	O	100–400 mg daily
Amikacin	Amikacin	Amikin	IV	15 mg/kg daily
Amiloride hydrochloride		Midamor	O	5–15 mg daily
Aminocaproic acid	Aminocaproic acid	Amicar, Epsikapron, Epsilon-amino-N-caproic acid	IV	5 g initially, 1·25 g/hr
Aminophylline	Aminophylline		R, IV	100–300 mg/dose
Amiodarone		Cordarone	IV	2–5 mg/kg over 0·5–3 min
Amoxycillin	Amoxicillin	Amoxil, Larotid, Polymox	O	0·2–1·2 g daily
Amphotericin	Amphotericin B	Fungizone	O	0·75–1·5 g daily
Ampicillin	Ampicillin	Omnipen, Penbritin, Polycillin	IV	0·25–1·0 mg/kg/day
Aspirin	Aspirin	Aspro, Disprin, Solprin	O, Inj	1–4 g daily
Atenolol		Tenormin	O, R	0·3–1·0 g 6-hourly
Atropine sulphate	Atropine sulfate		O	50–200 mg daily
			Inj	0·6–1·2 mg

Table 18 continued overleaf

293

Table 18 continued

British	American	Common proprietary names	Route	Usual adult dose
Bendrofluazide	Bendroflumethiazide	Aprinox, Benuron, Naturetin, Neo-Na Clex	O	2·5–10·0 mg daily
Benzathine penicillin	Penicillin G-Benzathine	Penidural LA, Bicillin LA	IM	1·2 mega units monthly
Benzylpenicillin	Penicillin G	Crystapen	Inj	2·4–12 g (4–20 mega units) daily
Betamethasone	Betamethasone	Betnesol, Celestone	O	0·5–16 mg daily
Bretylium tosylate	Bretylium tosylate	Bretylol	Inj	5–10 mg/kg every 2–8 hr
Calcium chloride	Calcium chloride		IV	5–10 mmol/dose
Calcium gluconate	Calcium gluconate	Calcium Sandoz (equiv.)	IV	5–20 ml of 10% solution/dose (1·1–4·5 mmol)
Captopril	Captopril	Capoten	O	25–50 mg thrice daily
Cefoxitin	Cefoxitin	Mefoxin	Inj	3–12 g daily
Cephradine	Cephradine	Anspor, Velosef	O	1–4 g daily
			IV	2–4 g daily
Cephalothin sodium	Cephalothin sodium	Keflin	Inj	2–6 g daily
Chloramphenicol	Chloramphenicol	Chloromycetin	O, Inj	1·5–3·0 g daily
Chlorhexidine	—	Hibitane	Local app	—
Chlorothiazide	Chlorothiazide	Chlotride, Diuril, Saluric	O	0·5–1·5 g daily
Chlorpromazine hydrochloride	Chlorpromazine hydrochloride	Largactil, Thorazine	O, Inj	25–50 mg/dose
Chlortetracycline hydrochloride	Chlortetracyline hydrochloride	Aureomycin	O	1–3 g daily
Clindamycin	Clindamycin	Dalacin C, Cleocin	O	0·6–1·2 g daily
Clindamycin		Dalacin C Phosphate	Inj	0·6–2·7 g daily

Approved name	Chemical name	Proprietary name	Route	Dose
Clonidine	Clonidine	Catapres	O IV	300–900 µg daily 2 µg/kg/dose
Cloxacillin sodium	Cloxacillin sodium	Orbenin, Tego-Pen	O, Inj	1·5–3·0 g daily
Cortisone acetate	Cortisone acetate	Compound E, Cortelan, Cortisyl, Cortogen, Cortone	O, IM	50–400 mg daily (short term) 12·5–50·0 mg daily (replacement)
Co-trimoxazole	Co-trimoxazole	Bactrim, Septrin Septra Cotrizol Bactrim, Septrin	O IV	1920 mg daily 1920–2880 mg daily
Crystal violet	—	Gentian violet	Local app	
Cyclopenthiazide	—	Navidrex	O	0·5–1·5 mg daily
Dexamethasone	Dexamethasone	Decadron, Oradexon Deksone	O, Inj	2–20 mg daily (bigger doses in, e.g. shock)
Diazepam	Diazepam	Valium	O Inj	4–40 mg daily 5–40 mg/dose
Diazoxide	Diazoxide	Hyperstat	IV	5 mg/kg, single dose
Digoxin	Digoxin	Lanoxin	O, Inj	see p. 109
Dipyridamole	Dipyridamole	Persantine, Persantin 100	O Inj	150–400 mg daily 10–30 mg daily
Disopyramide	Disopyramide	Norpace, Rythmodan (and Retard) Disopyramide Durule	O IV	200–600 mg daily 3 mg/kg, in 1 hr, then 0.4 mg/kg/hr
Dobutamine	Dobutamine	Dobutrex	IV	2·5–10 µg/kg/min
Dopamine	Dopamine HCl	Intropin	IV	1–10 µg/kg/min, rarely to 50 µg/kg/min
Ephedrine hydrochloride	Ephedrine sulfate		O Inj	15–60 mg 3–4 times daily 10–30 mg/dose

Table 18 continued overleaf

Table 18 continued

| Approved name | | Common proprietary names | Route | Usual adult dose |
British	American			
Erythromycin	Erythromycin	Emu-V, Erythrocin, Ilotycin	O, IV	1–2 g daily
Fenoterol		Berotec	Inhal	200–400 µg by aerosol
Flucloxacillin		Floxapen	O	0.75–1.5 g daily
Flucytosine	Flucytosine	Ancobon, Alcobon	O	100–200 mg/kg/day
			IV	150–200 mg/kg/day
Frusemide	Furosemide	Lasix, Frusid	O	20–40 mg/dose
			Inj	40–80 mg/dose
Gentamicin sulphate	Gentamicin sulfate	Cidomycin, Garamycin	Inj	3–5 mg/kg/day
Glyceryl trinitrate	Nitroglycerin	Anginine, Nitrostat Nitrolingual	O	0.3–0.9 mg sublingually
			IV	0.4–4 µg/per/min
	Nitroglycerin	Nitrobid, Nitrol, Nitrong	Topical	1–5 inches 2% ointment 4 hourly
Guanethidine sulphate	Guanethidine sulfate	Ismelin	O	5–10 mg initially, increasing to 300 mg daily
Heparin	Sodium heparin	Bioheprin, Hepathrom, Lipoheprin, Liquemin, Panheprin, Pularin	IV	5000–15 000 units/dose
Hexachlorophane	Hexachlorophene	Phisohex	Local app	
Hydralazine	Hydralazine	Apresoline, Rolazine, Dralzine	O	50–400 mg daily
			IV	0.05–0.3 mg/kg/dose
Hydrochlorothiazide	Hydrochlorothiazide	Esidrex, Hydro-diuril, Oretic	O	25–150 mg daily
Hydrocortisone sodium succinate	Hydrocortisone (cortisol)	Ef-cortelan soluble, Solucortef	Inj	0.3–1.0 g daily or as single dose

			Route	Dose
Iodophor	Iodophor	Betadine, Iodosan, Isodine, Wescodyne	Local app	
Isoprenaline hydrochloride	Isoproterenol hydrochloride	Isuprel	IV	0·05–0·5 μg/kg/min
Labetalol	Labetalol	Trandate	O	200–600 mg daily
Lignocaine hydrochloride	Lidocaine hydrochloride	Lidocaine	IV	50–200 mg
		Leostesin, Xylocaine, Xylocard	IV	see p. 112
Lorazepam	Lorazepam	Ativan	O	2–6 mg daily
Metaraminol Tartrate	Metaraminol bitartrate	Aramine, Pressonex	Inj	2–10 mg/dose
Methoxamine hydrochloride	Methoxamine hydrochloride	Vasoxine, Vasoxyl	Inj	2·50–20 mg/dose
Methyldopa	Methyldopa	Aldomet	O	0·5–2 g daily
Methylprednisolone	Methylprednisolone	Medrol	O	8–80 mg daily
Methylprednisolone sodium succinate	Methylprednisolone sodium succinate	Solu-medrol	IV	15–30 mg/kg (for shock)
Metoprolol	Metoprolol	Betaloc, Lopresor	O	100–200 mg daily
Metronidazole	Metronidazole	Flagyl	O	1·2 g daily
			IV	1·5 g daily
			R	3 g daily
Mexilitene	—	Mexitil	O	600–800 mg daily
			IV	250 mg in 10 min, 250 mg in 1 hr, 250 mg in 2 hr, then 0·5 mg–1 mg/min
Morphine sulphate	Morphine sulfate		Inj	5–20 mg/dose
Naloxone	Naloxone	Narcan	Inj	0·4 mg
Neomycin sulphate	Neomycin sulfate	Myciguent, Spersin	Local app	

Table 18 continued overleaf

Table 18 continued

Approved name — British	Approved name — American	Common proprietary names	Route	Usual adult dose
Neostigmine methylsulphate	Neostigmine methylsulfate	Prostigmin	Inj	0·5–5·0 mg/dose
Nitrazepam	—	Mogadon	O	5–10 mg/dose
Noradrenaline	Levarterenol	Levophed	IV	8–12 μg/min reducing to 2–4 μg /min
Nystatin	Nystatin	Nilstat, Mycostatin	O	0·5–1·0 mega units 3 times daily
Oxazepam	Oxazepam	Adumbran, Serepax, Serax	O	30–120 mg daily
Oxprenolol	Oxprenolol	Trasicor	O	60–480 mg daily
			Inj	1–2 mg/dose
Papaveretum	Opium alkaloids concentrated	Omnopon, Pantopan	Inj	10–20 mg/dose
Paraldehyde	Paraldehyde		IM, R	5–10 ml/dose
Pentazocine	Pentazocine	Fortral, Talwin	IM, O	30–60 mg/dose
Perhexiline		Pexid	O	200–400 mg daily
Pethidine hydrochloride	Meperidine	Demerol, Isonipecaine,	O, Inj	25–100 mg/dose
Phenobarbitone sodium	Phenobarbital sodium	Gardenal, Luminal	O	30–120 mg
			IM	100–200 mg
Phenoxybenzamine hydrochloride	Phenoxybenzamine hydrochloride	Dibenyline, Dibenzyline	IV	1 mg/kg over 1 hr
Phenoxymethylpenicillin	Pencillin V	Compocillin VK, Crystapen VK	O	1–4 g daily
Phentolamine mesylate	Phentolamine mesylate	Regitine, Rogitine	IV	2–30 μg/kg/min

Phenylephrine	Neosynephrine	IV	100–180 μg/min reducing to 40–60 μg/min
Phenytoin sodium	Danten, Denyl, Dilantin, Diphenylan, Epanutin	O	First dose 1 g
		O, Inj	50–400 mg daily
Phytomenadione	Aquamephyton, Konakion, Vitamin K₁	O, Inj	5–20 mg/dose
Pindolol	Visken	O	15–60 mg daily
		Inj	0·4 mg/dose
Polymyxin B sulphate	Polymyxin B sulfate	Local app	
Potassium chloride	Aerosporin Slow K, Span K, Sando K, Chlorvescent	O, IV	16–48 mmol daily
Prazosin	Minipress	O	3–20 mg daily
Prednisolone	Delta cortef, Sterane	O	10–100 mg daily
Prednisone	Deltasone, Meticorten, Deltacortelan	O	10–100 mg daily
Procainamide hydrochloride	Pronestyl	IV	up to 1 g slowly
		O	0·5–1·5 g/dose
Prochlorperazine maleate	Compazine, Stemetil	O, Inj	10–30 mg daily
		R	25–50 mg
Promethazine hydrochloride	Phenergan, Quadnite, Provigan, Z.Pam	O	25–75 mg daily
		Inj	20–50 mg daily
Propranolol	Inderal	O	30–600 mg daily
		IV	3–10 mg
Proscillaridin	Talusin	O	0·5–2·0 mg daily
Protamine sulphate	Protamine sulfate	Inj	1 mg counteracts 100 units of heparin
Quinidine sulphate	Quinidine sulfate Kinidin durules, Quiditard	O, Inj	see p. 112

Table 18 continued overleaf

Table 18 continued

Approved name British	Approved name American	Common proprietary names	Route	Usual adult dose
Reserpine	Reserpine	Serpasil	O	0·5–2·5 mg daily
			IM	0·1–0·5 mg/dose
Rolitetracycline		Reverin	IV	275–825 mg daily
Salbutamol	Albuterol	Ventolin	O	6–16 mg daily
			Inj	250 μg IV, 500 μg SC
			Inhal	100–200 μg by aerosol, repeated
Sodium Nitroprusside	Sodium Nitroprusside	Nipride	IV	0·5–8 μg/kg/min
Sodium polystyrene sulphonate	Sodium polystyrene sulfonate	Kayexalate, Resonium A	O	15–60 g daily
			R	25 g up to 12 times daily
Sorbide nitrate	Isosorbide dinitrate	Isordil, Isotrate, Carvasin	O	30–120 mg daily (5–10 mg sublingual)
Spironolactone	Spironolactone	Aldactone	O	100–200 mg daily
Streptomycin sulphate	Streptomycin sulfate	Strepolin	IM	0·5–1·0 g daily
Sulphadiazine	Sulfadiazine		O	2–4 g daily
Sulpadimidine	Sulfamethazine	Sulphamezathine	O	4–6 g daily
Sulphafurazole	Sulfisoxazole	Gantrisin, Sodizole, Sulphazole	O	4–6 g daily
Sulphinpyrazone	Sulfinpyrazone	Anturan	O	600–800 mg daily
Suxamethonium chloride	Succinylcholine chloride	Anectine, Sucostrin, Scoline	IV	30–100 mg

Terbutaline	Terbutaline sulfate	Bricanyl, Brethine	O Inj Inh	5–15 mg daily 250 μg 250–500 μg by aerosol, repeated
Tetracylcine	Tetracycline	Achromycin, Hostacycline Panmycin, Polycyline, Tetracyn	O	1–2 g daily
Theophylline	Theophylline	Bronkodyl, Nuelin (and SR) Theolair SR	O	0·5–1·0 g daily
Thiamine	Thiamine	Vitamin B$_1$	O, Inj	25–100 mg daily
Ticarcillin		Tarcil	IV	200–300 mg/kg/day
Tolazoline	Tolazoline	Priscol	IV	10–50 mg
Triamterene	Triamterene	Dyrenium, Dytac	O	150–250 mg daily
Trimeprazine	Trimeprazine	Temaril, Vallergan	O	10–40 mg daily
Trimetaphan camsylate	Trimethaphan	Arfonad	IV, drip	
Trometamol	Tromethamine	Tham, Tris-buffer	IV	0·3 mol in 1 hr 0·6 mol in 12 hr
Tubocurarine chloride	Tubocurarine chloride	Tubadil, Tubarine	IV	3 mg test dose 5–20 mg/dose
Verapamil	Verapamil	Isoptin	O IV	40–80 mg thrice daily 3–10 mg
Warfarin sodium	Sodium warfarin	Coumadin, Marevan, Panwarfin	O	3–10 mg daily

Appendix 3
Nutrition

Table 19 Estimated daily protein and caloric requirements for adult patients

	Protein (g)	Calories (kJ)
Preoperative (apyrexial)	45–75	1500–2000 (6·3–8·4)
Postoperative (uncomplicated)	75–125	2000–3500 (8·4–14·7)
Multiple injuries, major sepsis or burns	100–300	3500–5000 (14·7–21·0)

Energy requirements increase by 10–12% for each 1°C rise in temperature.

Table 20 *(facing page)* Approximate protein, fat, carbohydrate, sodium, potassium and iron content of various foods, with caloric value of 100 g of each.

Food	Protein (g per 100 g)	Fat (g per 100 g)	Carbohydrate	Sodium (mmol per 100 g)	Potassium (mmol per 100 g)	Iron (mg per 100 g)	Calories per 100 g	Kilojoules per 100 g
Bread, white	8·0	1·5	53	22	3	1·8	240	1004
Cornflakes	6·5	1·0	88	46	3	2·8	370	1548
Farex	13	2·5	73	12	8	24	350	1464
Rice, boiled	2·0	0·5	30	0·1	1	0·2	122	510
Butter	0·5	85	—	10	0·5	0·2	790	3300
Cheese, Wensleydale	29	31	—	16	5	0·3	406	1698
Cow's milk, whole	3·5	3·5	5·0	2	4	0·1	66	276
Human milk	2·0	3·5	7·0	2	2	0·1	68	284
Egg, whole	12	13	—	6	4	2·5	163	682
Beef, sirloin, roast	22	32	—	3	7	4·5	385	1611
Chicken, boiled	26	11	—	4	10	2·0	203	849
Mutton, leg, roast	25	21	—	3	9	4·5	292	1222
Flounder, steamed	20	1·5	—	5	8	1·5	95	397
Oysters, shelled	10	1·0	—	22	7	6·0	50	209
Trout, steamed	23	4·5	—	4	10	1·0	133	556
Apples	0·5	—	12	0·1	3	0·3	47	197
Bananas	1·0	—	19	0·05	9	0·4	77	322
Grapes	0·5	—	16	0·1	6	0·3	63	263
Melons	1·0	—	5·3	0·5	8	0·8	24	100
Oranges	1·0	—	8·5	0·1	5	0·3	35	146
Cabbage, boiled	1·5	—	1·0	0·5	3	0·7	9	38
Carrots, boiled	0·5	—	4·5	2	2	0·4	19	79
Peas, boiled	5·0	—	7·5	—	4	1·2	49	205
Potatoes, boiled	1·5	—	20	0·1	8	0·5	80	335
Swedes, boiled	1·0	—	4·0	0·5	3	0·3	18	75
Horlick's milk powder	15	8	71	30	29	1·5	399	1669

Table 21 Approximate analysis of milk and artificial feeds (per 1000 Calorie (4·2 kJ) equivalent).

	Volume (ml)	Powder (g)	Protein (g)	Carbo-hydrate (g)	Fat (g)	Sodium (mmol)	Potassium (mmol)
Cow's milk	1480	–	50·3	69·6	57·8	36·8	58·2
Human milk	1470	–	30·4	102·9	51·5	11·5	20·2
Cream	276	–	5·8	8·3	105·0	7·8	16·1
SMA	1525	193	22·9	106·9	53·4	16·8	29·0
Enfamil	1492	190	22·8	103·6	55·1	14·5	29·6
Complan		226	37·3	131·2	36·2	31·0	39·4
Thrive		282	67·4	178·5	1·6	40·1	87·1
Flexical		226	22·6	153·2	34·1	15·7	31·9
Vivonex		266	20·4	225·8	1·4	37·3	29·9
Vivonex HN		226	41·5	209·8	0·9	33·4	17·9

In the usual concentration milk mixtures contain about 0·67 Calories (2·8 kJ) per ml. Most of the artificial feeds contain about 1 Calorie (4·2 kJ) per ml but this can be changed to suit the volume requirements of a patient. It is wise to use diluted solutions when introducing a feed.

Table 22 An example of a solution for adult total parenteral nutrition.

Freamine II 8·5%	1500 ml	
Dextrose 50% in water	1500 ml	
Sodium	135 mmol	
Potassium	121 mmol	Made up in a single 3 l unit.
Magnesium	12 mmol	
Chloride	100 mmol	
Acetate	120 mmol	
Phosphate	60 mmol	
Insulin	As required	

Trace Elements (per day)

Zinc	4 mg
Copper	1·5 mg
Manganese	20 µg
Chromium	10 µg
Iodide	100 µg
Selenium	50 µg

Multivitamin injection, Folic acid 1 mg IM daily
Vitamin K 10 mg IM weekly
Vitamin B_{12} IM as required
Intralipid 10% or 20% 500 ml twice weekly by peripheral administration

Appendix 4
Some Normal Values

Haemaglobin	120–160 g/litre
White cell count	$4.0–10.0 \times 10^9$/litre
Platelets	$150–400 \times 10^9$/litre
Whole blood clotting time	4–10 min
Therapeutic range	20–25 min
Prothrombin ratio	0·8–1·2
Therapeutic range	2·0–4·0
Activated partial thromboplastin time	25–35 seconds
Urea	4·0–7·0 mmol/litre
Creatinine	0·05–0·11 mmol/litre
Sodium	135–146 mmol/litre
Potassium	3·5–5·0 mmol/litre
Calcium	2·10–2·55 mmol/litre
Magnesium	0·8–1·0 mmol/litre
Random glucose	4·0–9·0 mmol/litre
pH	7·35–7·45
P_{CO_2}	5–6 kPa (35–45 mmHg)
P_{O_2}	11–13 kPa (80–100 mmHg)
Base excess	± 2·5 mmol/litre
Bicarbonate	18–23 mmol/litre
O_2 saturation	95–100 per cent
Plasma haemoglobin	0–100 mg/litre

Appendix 5

Electrical Hazards in the ICU

A great deal of electrical apparatus is used in the ICU, and staff must know how electrical hazards can be minimized. Fatal ventricular fibrillation may occur if a current is accidentally passed through the heart, and there is some risk of this unless strict rules are observed.

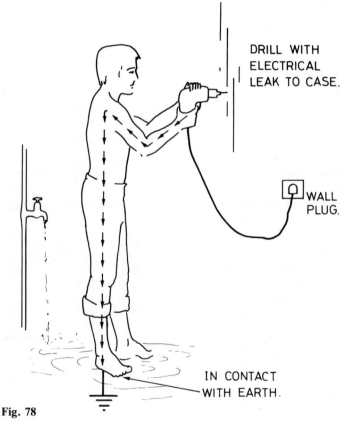

DRILL WITH ELECTRICAL LEAK TO CASE.

WALL PLUG.

IN CONTACT WITH EARTH.

Fig. 78

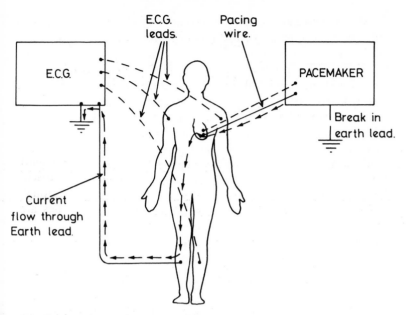

Fig. 79

The mains voltage is 230 volts (in some countries, 110 volts). The dry body has a high resistance to current flow — say 100 000 ohms. If the mains socket or an exposed, live wire is touched, there is only a small flow of current through the body even if there is a free contact with earth. Using the above examples, current = voltage/resistance = 230/100 000 = 2·3 milliamperes, enough to cause a shock but not ventricular fibrillation. If, on the other hand, the body is immersed in water and the water earthed, resistance may be reduced to, say 1000 ohms and the current would be 230 mA, which is quite enough to cause ventricular fibrillation.

A minor fault in electrical equipment can cause leakage of electricity to the case surrounding it. Handling mains-operated equipment while standing in water can therefore cause ventricular fibrillation (Fig. 79). An earth lead, for instance the right leg lead in the ordinary ECG connection, also provides free conduction to earth. No patient connected with an earth lead should therefore handle any mains-operated electrical apparatus — shaver, hair dryer, radio, television set, etc.

Most patients are connected at some time with more than one set of electrical apparatus, e.g. pressure-monitoring apparatus and ECG. To guard against accidents, electrical isolating circuits and earthing cables are commonly used, but no system can be considered permanently faultless and regular checks are essential. Special risk arises from any equipment in direct contact with the heart, such as pacing wires. In the arrangement shown in Fig. 79, a fault in the earthing of either the pacemaker or the ECG machine could lead to the passage of current through the heart and in this setting very small currents may cause ventricular fibrillation. For this reason, *battery-operated external pacemakers* (with no connection to the mains or earth) *are always used when the patient is connected with any electrical apparatus.* Even a cannula in an artery or vein carries the risk of passing current through the heart; fortunately, this is not as high as with pacemaker wires applied directly to the myocardium or with catheters extending into the cardiac chambers.

Appendix 6
SI Units of Pressure

The application of Système Internationale (SI) units in medicine is well advanced in European countries and some others. So far as this book is concerned, two units merit comment.

1 *Units of concentration* are to be molar, that is mol per l or mmol per l. These units replace Eq and mEq (see p. 6) and are intended to replace also g, mg and percentage units. Thus 5 per cent glucose (5 g per 100 ml) will become 278 mmol per l, since the molecular weight of glucose is 180. For the present we have replaced only Eq and mEq and have retained mosm (p. 92).

2 *Units of pressure* are the Pascal (Pa) and the kiloPascal (kPa), where 1 mm Hg = 0·133 kPa. These units are to apply to all pressure measurements except (quite illogically) blood pressure. The latter will continue to be expressed in mmHg but the resistance unit derived from it (see p. 50) will be based on pressure in kPa and blood flow in l per second — again, this seems quite illogical. In this book we have given blood pressures in mmHg and for all other pressures have given approximate equivalents in both mmHg and kPa. Table 23 is a ready reckoner for conversion from one unit to the other.

3 The SI unit of energy is the kilojoule (kJ); 4·184 kJ = 1 kilocalorie (Cal, p. 20).

Appendix 6

Table 23 Conversion of pressure units.

mmHg	kPa	kPa	mmHg
10	1·33	1	7·50
20	2·67	2	15·00
30	4·00	3	22·50
40	5·33	4	30·00
50	6·67	5	37·50
60	8·00	6	45·00
70	9·33	7	72·50
80	10·67	8	60·00
90	12·00	9	67·50
100	13·33	10	75·00
200	26·66	20	150·00
300	40·00	30	225·00
400	53·33	40	300·00
500	66·66	50	375·00
600	79·99	60	450·00
700	93·33	70	525·00

Recommended Reading

Intensive Care — General Texts

ABELS, LINDA F. (1979) *Mosby's Manual of Critical Care*. C. V. Mosby, St. Louis.

ADLER, DIANE C. & SHOEMAKER, NORMA J. (eds.) (1979) *AACN (American Association of Critical Care Nurses), Organisation & Management of Critical Care Facilities*. C. V. Mosby, St. Louis.

HAMILTON, ARDITH J. (1981) *Critical Care Nursing Skills*. Appleton-Century-Crofts, New York.

HAZZARD, MARY E. (1978) *Critical Care Nursing*. Medical Examination, Garden City.

HOLLOWAY, NANCY M. (1979) *Nursing the Critically Ill Adult*. Addison-Wesley, Menlo Park, California.

HUDAK, CAROLYN M. *et al.* (1977) *Critical Care Nursing*, 2nd edn. Lippincott, Philadelphia.

KENNER, CORNELA V., GUZETTA, CATHIE E., DOSSEY, BARBARA M. (1980) *Critical Care Nursing: Mind-Body-Spirit*. Little Brown, Boston.

KINNEY, MARGUERITE RODGERS *et al.* (1980) *AACN's Clinical Reference for Critical Care Nursing*. McGraw-Hill, New York.

TINKER J. & PORTER S.W. (1980) *A Course in Intensive Therapy Nursing*. Edward Arnold, London.

Physiology

LUCIANO, DOROTHY *et al.* (1978) *Human Function & Structure*. McGraw-Hill, New York.

GREEN J.H. (1969) *Basic Clinical Physiology*. University Press, Oxford.

Ischaemic Heart Disease

ANDREOLI, KATHLEEN G. *et al.* (1975) *Comprehensive Cardiac Care — a text for nurses, physicians and other health practitioners*, 3rd edn. C. V. Mosby, St. Louis.

CROMWELL, RUE L. *et al.* (1977) *Acute Myocardial Infarction: Reaction & Recovery*. C. V. Mosby, St. Louis.

FARDY P.S. *et al.* (1979) *Cardiac Rehabilitation — implications for the nurse and other health professionals.* C. V. Mosby, St. Louis.

MELTZER E. & DUNNING J. (1972) *Textbook of Coronary Care.* Charles Press, Bowie, Maryland.

OLIVER M.F., JULIAN D.G., BROWN, MYRA G. (1974) *Intensive Coronary Care.* WHO, Geneva.

GENTRY W.D. & WILLIAMS R.B. JR. (eds.) (1979) *Psychological Aspects of Myocardial Infarction & Coronary Care*, 2nd edn. C. V. Mosby, St. Louis.

Cardiac Surgery

BRAIMBRIDGE M.V. (1981) *Post-operative Cardiac Intensive Care*, 3rd edn. Blackwell Scientific Publications, Oxford.

FLEMING J.S. & BRAIMBRIDGE M.V. (1974) *Lecture Notes on Cardiology*, 2nd edn. Blackwell Scientific Publications, Oxford.

JACKLE, MARY & HALLIGAN, MARNEY (1980) *Cardiovascular Problems: A Critical Care Nursing Focus.* Brady, Bowie, Maryland.

KING O. (1975) *Care of the Cardiac Surgical Patient.* C. V. Mosby, St. Louis.

SADE R.M. *et al.* (1977) *Infant & Child Care in Heart Surgery.* Year Book, Chicago.

PETTY T.L. (1976) *Intensive & Rehabilitative Respiratory Care*, 2nd edn. Lea & Febiger, Philadelphia.

RAREY K.P. & YOUTSEY J.W. (1978) *Respiratory Patient Care.* Prentice Hall, Englewood Cliffs, New Jersey.

Neonatal

KLAUS M.H. & FANAROFF A.A. (1973) *Care of the High-Risk Neonate.* W.B. Saunders, Philadelphia.

CRAIG W.S. *et al.* (1969) *Care of the Newly Born Infant*, 4th edn. Churchill Livingstone, Edinburgh.

HARPER, RITA G. & YOON, JING JA (1976) *Handbook of Neonatology.* Year Book, Chicago.

CHISWICK M.L. (1978) *Neonatal Medicine.* Update, London.

Index